Waiting ON PINS AND NEEDLES

Different Paths to Parenthood Through the Eyes of a Fertility Acupuncturist

RACHEL BLUNK, LAC, FABORM

Copyright © 2021 by Rachel Blunk, LAc, FABORM.

All rights reserved. No part of this book may be reproduced in any written, electronic, recording, or photocopying without written permission of the publisher or author. The exception would be in the case of brief quotations embodied in articles or reviews and pages where permission is specifically granted by the publisher or author.

Rachel Blunk, LAc, FABORM/Waiting on Pins and Needles
Printed in the United States of America

Although every precaution has been taken to verify the accuracy of the information contained herein, the author and publisher assume no responsibility for any errors or omissions. No liability is assumed for damages that may result from the use of information contained within.

Waiting on Pins and Needles/ Rachel Blunk, LAc, FABORM -- 1st ed.

ISBN 9798500593290 Print Edition

CONTENTS

Foreword vii

Introduction xl

Preface 1

Recurrent Miscarriage: Flight of the Unborn Angels 7

Fourth Time's a Charm: My Story 9

Itching to Conceive 17

Nevertheless, She Persisted 23

Uterine Anomalies: A "Unicornuate" Uterus? 33

Double Trouble 35

Against All Odds 41

IVF: Test Tube Babies 49

The Gift of Life 51

Running Low on Eggs: Low Anti-Müllerian Hormone 59

Past the Expiration Date 61

Advanced Maternal Age: Too Old to Have Children? 65

Sperm Hats and Eggs on Ice 67

East Meets West in Fertility Treatment 71

Ancient Chinese Medicine Secret 75

Unexplained Fertility: Unsolved Fertility Mysteries 81

Sister Secrets 83

When the Time is Right 93

Egg Donation: Borrowed Eggs 97

Donor Egg IVF Virgin 99

Triple Treasure 105

The Perfect Banana 111

Embryo Adoption: Snowflake Adoption 119

Snowflake Baby 121

Egg Donation: The Giving Eggs 127

Is Something Wrong with My Eggs? 129

The Great Giveaway 133

Adoption: Babies from the Heart 137

More Beautiful Than We Can Imagine 139

Surrogacy: Womb for Rent 145

A Beautiful Arrangement 147

Pregnancy and Infant Loss: When Things Go Wrong 153

Every Part of My Soul 155

Unbroken Courage 161

Ovarian Rebellion 169

The Courage to Try Again 175

Glossary 183

Acknowledgments 191

About the Author 193

Resources 195

*This is dedicated to Njemile Carol Jones, LAc, FABORM.
A beautiful soul inside and out, she was my classmate, colleague,
friend and birthday buddy.*

FOREWORD

It's time…

We're ready. Our entire relationship has been dedicated to preventing getting pregnant. We've finished school, we're in a relationship, we've got a job and a secure home. IT'S TIME!! What do we do? Just stop preventing and it will happen. Taking a prenatal vitamin will help. This is exciting and will be fun!

Six months later…

This was supposed to be easy. It should have happened by now. What are we doing wrong? Are we stressed? Is there a problem? Is the timing right? Let's do some research.

Ovulation predictor kits. I modified my diet. Take a "better" prenatal vitamin. Lose the briefs - here are your boxers. Check out sex positions that make babies. Lay in bed 30 minutes after sex with my feet in the air. Stop caffeine and drop the alcohol. Track my cycle on an app so I know exactly when it should happen. Keep trying - these methods will work. I've googled every method that may help - pineapple core, a lubricant, supplements. Let's try these. I'm feeling more resolved because this will work.

Twelve months later…

Frustration has turned to desperation. Will we be able to have kids? Can this happen? There is a problem. We need help. Sex isn't fun any more. I don't want to do it when the kit says I should. My partner is losing interest and we're fighting about it - all the time. Maybe I should try my primary care doctor and get some tests. Maybe my ob/gyn can help figure this out. I need a sperm test. Is our relationship strong enough for this? Does my insurance cover what comes next? Who do we see - my regular doctor, an acupuncturist, a naturopath, an ob/gyn, a nutritionist, a fertility specialist, all or none of the above?

One in eight couples will experience issues with fertility. What starts off as a simple plan quickly morphs into a complicated science experiment wrapped in a hurricane of emotions. The pathway that leads to a family varies for every person and couple. Because there are many causes, there are many approaches to reach the solution.

It is gut wrenching to begin the journey. It requires admitting there is a problem. An event that is usually kept between a couple becomes open to outsiders. You are part of a group you didn't know existed and don't want to join. A team that you never wanted is now reviewing your most personal and intimate moments. It is difficult, embarrassing, frustrating, sad, and annoying. As has been said, the first step is the hardest.

You have to find the right team to invite into your life. The goal is a short, intense, emotional relationship to help you navigate your options to conceive. Your team can consist of members from varied backgrounds. Each professional mentioned above brings a benefit of experience and treatment options. Many offer more natural methods to optimize your fertility while others can be more aggressive medical choices.

The team you select should work together in a complementary way to enhance your fertility. It shouldn't increase your stress, make it hard or be divisive. Each specialty can bring unique aspects to your care and the focus should be you. The best approach is to let you drive the car deciding the ultimate speed and direction you take while your team holds the map, gives you fuel and keeps the engine humming.

In my nearly twenty years as a fertility physician, I have had the honor and privilege of working with many amazing and instrumental fertility providers including Rachel Blunk, the author of this inspiring book. Rachel is a powerful force guiding patients through their journey of becoming a family. Alone, and as a wonderful complement to traditional medical care, her acupuncture skills have helped countless couples become parents. Traditional needles and remedies aside, she is also a friend, counselor, and shoulder to lean on during difficult times for fertility patients.

In this book you will have insight into the world of fertility care. The struggles, journeys, sadness, and victories emanate from decades of being a consummate professional. Rachel compassionately realizes the elation and heartbreak from her pivotal role in creating families, caring for her patients and being a true friend in times of need. I hope you enjoy her insightful view into this world of infertility, where one in eight couples unwittingly find themselves. If you do happen to find yourself in this world, it is a comfort to know Rachel will be on your team.

Dr Robert Gustofson, M.D. FACOG, of the Colorado Center for Reproductive Medicine

INTRODUCTION

As a fertility acupuncturist living and working in northern Colorado for nearly 20 years, I'd heard of Rachel's practice, Baby by Blunk, through the mouths of many satisfied patients for, what felt like, ever. And yet, even though we were practically in each other's backyards, we didn't meet until years later at a fertility conference in Vancouver, BC. We became fast friends and have since come to rely on each other as a source of wisdom, camaraderie, and support.

What I've come to learn in the years since is that Rachel is a gift—not just to me, but to our profession, and most certainly, to her patients. In addition to having a veritable wellspring of knowledge and experience, she also possesses an authentic presence that conveys genuine humility and care to all she meets. It is from this place that Rachel works with her patients, holding the space for each of them with tender care and understanding. It is a gift that we can all aspire to emulate.

In Waiting on Pins and Needles, we are invited into the realm of her astute wit and brave storytelling. This collection of stories gathered from her years of treating patients struggling with infertility shines a light on the perils and pitfalls—as well as the joys—that accompany many on the road to parenthood. Let it serve as a buoy and a comfort to those that follow in their footsteps.

Maren Cahill, DAOM, LAc, FABORM

PREFACE

During the months I treated Alana, her story kept coming up in my mind at the grocery store, while at the gym, while on walks. My brain thought her story was so amazing that it kept trying to burst forth from me. I finally sat down and wrote it, then asked her if it was okay that I had done that. She was more than delighted to have me share it, as she had also been blogging about it herself.

After getting Alana's story down on paper (well, in my computer), Elizabeth's story wouldn't leave me. Her tragedy was almost too much to bear, but she persevered anyway, in the face of huge obstacles as well as overwhelming grief. I felt I had to write it down as well.

After writing these stories down, I went through my patient files to see what others I could write. For hours, while leafing through old charts, I was brought right back to the treatment room with these women I had treated years before. I remembered past conversations with them: listening to their grief around infertility and humor around the awkwardness of their sex lives while trying to conceive is just so incredibly intimate. I felt honored that they would share these stories with me so honestly and in the raw.

Waiting on Pins and Needles is a collection of real stories about real patients I've seen in my clinic over the past 20 years, during which I've specialized in fertility acupuncture. Every woman in this book was generously willing to share her fertility journey, though some opted to remain anonymous—their names and other parts of their stories have been altered for anonymity. While some patients' identifying details have been changed for their privacy, others preferred to bare it all. Some stories are happy, and some tragic, but the common thread is that to me they are all fascinating in some way, whether a triplet pregnancy or persevering after the loss of a child. Fertility acupuncture isn't just about darling, chubby babies; it's also about heartbreak and tears along the way.

I am deeply grateful to the thousands of patients who have shared their most personal stories with me. Not everyone wants to discuss the gory details of their menstrual flow or the intimate details of their sex lives. When talking to people who aren't patients, I try to remember this, so I don't ask embarrassing questions.

One of the best perks of my job is being among the first to know that a woman is pregnant. To have her share that confidence with me, sometimes even before her husband or partner knows, is one of the best feelings in the world.

My own fertility struggles drew me to fertility acupuncture. My husband and I got pregnant and miscarried three times in a row. It was a long and miserable nine months before my body would let me get pregnant again, so I threw myself into figuring out how to fix it with acupuncture and Chinese herbs.

Thus began my passion for treating infertility. It was a difficult time for me personally, but the experience allows me to share a deeper understanding of the challenge each patient faces.

Chinese fertility medicine looks at the whole person instead of just their reproductive organs. We look at diet, exercise, and emotional health. I ask questions like, "How long is it between your menstrual cycles? Do you have cramps? Do you run hot or cold? What about at night? How's your sleep? Your sex drive? Your digestion?" The answers give me valuable information about a woman's fertility. I must remind myself to explain to them why treating their cold hands or digestive issues will positively affect their fertility. Otherwise, they might wonder, *why is she curious about whether or not I have gas? I'm here to have a baby.*

During a treatment, after getting the facts about a woman's cycle, I enjoy sitting and talking with her about her life. It helps me to understand other things that might be going on.

Sometimes, I don't know what to do with a case. When that happens, I ask my colleagues, other fertility acupuncturists who are certified by the American Board of Oriental Reproductive Medicine (ABORM), for help. We have lively, daily email discussions. (If you decide to see a fertility acupuncturist, try to find a practitioner who has this certification, so you can benefit from the help of someone with loads of extra training.) I also look back through my notes from the Integrative Fertility Symposium that I attend yearly in Vancouver, Canada. This symposium touches on all aspects of female and male fertility from the most basic to the most complicated, from both a Western and Eastern point of view.

Working in the field of fertility can be tough because patients don't typically come to me when things are going well. Some wonder how I deal with the grief and disappointment my clients face. I'm always optimistic that a patient can get pregnant. I've seen it happen so many times with women who have been trying from six months to six years—even with the stories that seem the most hopeless.

It's almost never hopeless for a woman who wants to have a baby. The only time I said "no" to treating a potential client was when approached by a 47-year-old woman already in menopause whose husband had had a vasectomy. In that case, there were too many obstacles to overcome, so I referred her to a fertility doctor. I once helped prepare a 58-year-old woman for in vitro fertilization (IVF) who went on to have two children using donor eggs, her husband's sperm, and her own uterus. I doubt doctors would allow a woman of her age to attempt that today, but at the time, it was incredible.

If the male partner has vigorous, plentiful sperm and the female partner has healthy eggs, open tubes, and a sound uterus, pregnancy can happen. And if they aren't in good shape at the moment, acupuncture and herbs can address that. If all else fails, for example in cases of severe premature ovarian failure or a complete lack of sperm, the field of reproductive medicine creates miracles every day. The combination of Western and Eastern medicine for fertility is unbeatable.

When things go wrong, like when a patient miscarries, I always grieve for her. Miscarriages can be shocking and disheartening. But all is not lost. The sperm and egg found each other and implanted in the woman's uterus, so she is 50 percent there! The only times I've felt defeated were when patients have lost a full-term baby. This doesn't happen often, but when it does, it is truly devastating. These women are incredibly courageous because most want to jump right back into trying again.

My practice has changed me as a person and practitioner. Going to work with a focus on helping people instantly shifts me out of my head. It's so easy to ruminate over my own issues or the world's problems. Being engaged at work stops my navel-gazing and helps focus my attention on helping people achieve their dreams of starting or building a family. I can hardly think of a more rewarding line of work.

This isn't a how-to book. There are plenty of those types of books on the market. My intention is to give hope to women who may have lost it along the way and to provide stories for them to relate to. As Annie said about her own story, which is included in this book, "My husband and I really have no secrets. You can spill it all if you need to. We believe our story is not meant to be kept quiet. We have learned so much from listening to others, and we hope we can inspire others to not give up. It really is the biggest blessing when your child is finally placed in your arms, and you get to watch them grow and learn new things daily."

RECURRENT MISCARRIAGE: FLIGHT OF THE UNBORN ANGELS

A miscarriage is the loss of a viable pregnancy before 20 weeks, often due to genetic issues. Other causes include hormonal or thyroid imbalances, poor egg or sperm quality, and blood-clotting disorders, among others. According to the Mayo Clinic, about 10 to 20 percent of known pregnancies end in miscarriage. The actual number is likely higher because many miscarriages occur so early in pregnancy that a woman doesn't realize she's pregnant.

Miscarriage robs an expectant mother of the innocence of a first pregnancy. A woman who miscarries for the first time had never considered all the things that could go wrong until they did. The future hopes and dreams a woman places on the baby growing in her womb are lost when she miscarries. Women fear that the next one might not make it, and often aren't able to relax about their pregnancies until the end of the first trimester, or at least until they pass the week marker of their previous loss(es). Some women struggle with miscarriage anxiety through the entire pregnancy, until a successful delivery.

FOURTH TIME'S A CHARM: MY STORY

At first, my husband Scott and I thought we had it easy. We were blessedly naïve to the world of infertility. I was in my second year of practice as an acupuncturist and did not know much about fertility, yet. I was still treating mostly pain. At 31, I got pregnant the first time we tried! I thought, *this is easy!* Five weeks later, I miscarried. I was stunned, but we got right back on that horse and got pregnant again on the very next ovulation. Once again, I hardly made it to five weeks. I cried, but I didn't panic, not yet. I knew that at least the sperm and egg could find each other and implant.

I took herbs, sought acupuncture treatment, and we tried again. A couple of months later, I got pregnant very quickly with fraternal twins! Scott and I didn't expect twins, as they don't run in our families, but I was over the moon and, I must admit, a little apprehensive at the thought of caring for two infants at once. We showed the ultrasound photo to our parents, and they were thrilled.

When I had some spotting at around six weeks, I went to the OB's office for an ultrasound. The doctor told us that the first baby's heart had stopped beating. I was stunned and deeply sad but encouraged that the second baby's heart was still beating. We clung to the hope that the remaining twin would be okay. I went back the next week and learned that at seven weeks, the second one's heart had also stopped. Scott and I were devastated. When I did the math, it was bleak. Three pregnancies lost in five months. I was starting to worry that something was wrong with me.

I had told *everyone* that I was pregnant again and now had to tell *everyone* that I wasn't. It was horrible to have to repeat the words, "I lost the pregnancy." Each time I shared the news and saw the look in people's eyes, my sadness deepened. Friends brought flowers, sent cards, and told me their stories of miscarriage. This opened up a whole new world of fertility struggles. I had no idea that so many women miscarried. In fact, according to WebMD, 15-25 percent of all recognized pregnancies end in miscarriage. Up to 50 percent of pregnancies end in miscarriage before a woman even realizes she is pregnant and has missed her period. I didn't want to learn this the hard way, but it was reassuring to know I was not alone.

I wanted to pass the pregnancy naturally, but my OB advised against it because there would be a lot to pass with two embryos. For my mental health and physical comfort, she suggested a D&C. She was right. The recovery was much less painful physically than the previous two miscarriages.

After the D&C, it seemed that I couldn't get pregnant again. Whereas before, I got pregnant immediately, now my body didn't seem to want to get pregnant. These were the longest and most miserable nine months of my life.

I threw all my energy into figuring out how to heal myself with acupuncture and Chinese herbs and continued to see my own acupuncturist. I learned that I have two copies of the methyltetrahydrofolate reductase (MTHFR) gene mutation. People with the MTHFR gene mutation don't process the synthetic form of folate, called folic acid, correctly. This mutation can often lead to multiple miscarriages for women prone to this (like me). Whether or not the MTHFR gene mutation affects miscarriage is still debated in old-school circles in the fertility world. However, I took my functional MD's advice and switched to a prenatal vitamin with folate instead of folic acid.

In my practice, I've seen that when women who have had multiple miscarriages switch to folate, they often have successful pregnancies. *Is it the folate or the acupuncture?* It can be hard to tell. Still, it certainly doesn't hurt to switch to folate, as babies whose mothers have taken folate are also protected from neural tube defects, such as spina bifida. These days, most fertility doctors are aware of the folate/folic acid issue and preemptively put their patients on folate from the start. My patients take the dosage of folate that fertility doctors recommend. Switching to folate from folic acid is an easy, harmless, and inexpensive fix.

During the long and unexpected waiting period to get pregnant again, I pursued dreams that had been on my bucket list, intentionally choosing ones that would be challenging if I were pregnant or had a newborn. I traveled solo to Iceland for a week where I saw minke whales, hiked on a glacier, rode Icelandic horses, and soaked in the Blue Lagoon. I took lessons and learned to play the cello, something I had always wanted to do. When I had joined the orchestra as a sixth grader, I had been nudged into playing the viola since they were always short of violists. I liked the viola, but I had always secretly loved the cello.

I trained for and competed in a sprint mini triathlon, something I didn't think I could do. I don't recall my results, but I didn't come in last! And as an ex-synchronized swimmer, I beat most of the hardcore athletes out of the water. Of course, they zoomed past me during the bike and run segments, but I felt glory for a fleeting moment when I got out of the water before they did. I signed up for another triathlon in Glenwood Springs, Colorado. But, lo and behold, I had the happy task of writing to the race organizer to cancel my registration and get a refund because I learned I was pregnant for the fourth time. She refunded and congratulated me.

While I was super excited to be pregnant again, I was an anxious mess. This time, I protected myself and didn't tell anyone, so I wouldn't have to tell them when I would most likely eventually miscarry again. At an early ultrasound, around six weeks, we saw a strong heartbeat. I told the doctor I was spotting again (even though I wasn't) to get another ultrasound at seven weeks. The embryo was even bigger, and the heartbeat stronger. This was so much different than any of my previous pregnancies. When I finally made it past 12 weeks, I felt I was able to exhale completely. It seemed like this one might just work! I was nauseated in the first trimester and indeed complained about it, but I was thankful every day for the sign indicating the pregnancy was still good. The second and third trimesters were carefree and fun. I felt good and finally looked pregnant—not just like I had scarfed down all the cookies and pies over the winter holidays.

I was beyond grateful that the pregnancy went smoothly, and I anticipated a natural, drug-free delivery. Sadly, that dream was dashed because Calvin was in fetal distress, and I had an emergency C-section. In the end, though, I was just grateful that I had delivered a healthy, beautiful baby. As an added bonus, C-section babies are extra pretty because their heads aren't squished from squeezing through the birth canal. Just like my fertility struggles, not having the delivery I had hoped for has helped me better understand my patients' experiences.

Bringing Calvin home felt overwhelming. Filled with emotions that we had actually done it this time, I cried with relief and joy to finally have a baby in my arms. But I quickly realized that my miscarriage worries were relatively minor compared to bearing the responsibility for keeping a baby alive. How could the hospital in good conscience let me take this baby home? If something bad happened to him, it would be my fault. A whole new world of fears opened up for me. I had no idea how to care for a baby and he didn't come with an instruction manual. Unlike so many other women, I had almost never babysat! The internet wasn't really a thing yet, so I had to rely on books, instinct, Scott, and the advice of friends. Fortunately, he survived and thrived. But postpartum anxiety is no joke.

When Calvin was only nine months old, I was nursing him, and he pulled his head back and stared up at me in baby horror. I worried: *What's wrong? Does my milk taste weird? Is it something I ate?* I'll never forget his expression. He went on a nursing strike after that. I was perplexed but pumped for him at 40 ounces a day—my superpower. Weirdly, he was happy to take my milk from the bottle. Kids always seem to prefer packaged food. And mine was no different. Slowly, my supply dwindled to the point at which, two months later, I could only pump about four ounces a day. I was confused and sad until I started to feel nauseated in the morning and finally figured out what was going on. I was pregnant again! Calvin must have tasted the difference in my milk because of my pregnancy hormones and knew I was pregnant before I did. He's still a picky eater.

With my history, I was sure that my fifth pregnancy wouldn't stick. Week after week, I tried to quiet my anxious nerves, all the while anticipating a miscarriage. Four weeks turned into eight weeks, then sixteen. And six months into nine. It seemed that while in utero, Claire tried to keep my spirits light. When I was about eight months pregnant and my belly could rest on my thighs, she would reach her little hands above her head and move them, tickling my thighs. I jumped the first time I felt it! Then I thought, what a clever little one entertaining her mama. After I figured out what she was doing, I actually looked forward to it. It was the first of many delightful mother-daughter moments.

Just over 18 months after Calvin was born by C-section, baby Claire was born. My nurse-midwife was 100 percent confident that I could have a vaginal birth after C-section (VBAC), and she was right. Claire's head was in the 50th percentile (not too big) and was in the correct position for delivery. What a healing and wonderful experience to know that my lady parts worked properly, and I could get a baby out the old-fashioned way. Once again, I did not have the natural, drug-free birth I expected, and as a person in the natural healthcare field, I felt a little ashamed that I couldn't do it.

But honestly, the epidural was a little slice of heaven, and I wasn't getting a medal for having a natural birth anyway. My baby girl was perfect, and I didn't care how she came out, so long as she was healthy.

My fertility struggles were painful and difficult, but these experiences allow me to understand my patients' struggles. I don't know if I would have the depth of compassion and understanding if I hadn't gone through multiple miscarriages and then a nine-month bout of infertility. We all have our own stories. My fertility journey led to two beautiful, healthy children and an extremely rewarding career helping couples with infertility.

ITCHING TO CONCEIVE

"I'm doing everything I'm supposed to—eating one hundred percent organic, not drinking, not smoking, exercising, and yet, God or the universe or whoever's in charge isn't giving me a baby," said Kristi, a new patient, clearly frustrated. Thin and wiry with wavy brown hair and blue eyes, she was incensed. Many of my patients come in sad and grieving, but Kristi had moved past grief and was now fully into anger. This was a common and understandable state among patients. I had seen it many times before.

Kristi frowned and crossed her arms and legs in a harumph position. "I mean, if I'm not going to have a baby, I might as well be able to have some fun. You know?"

I laughed. "Yes, I do. Well, obviously, you're doing everything right, so there's something more going on. Let's see if we can get to the bottom of it."

"At thirty-seven and having been at this for five years, I won't lie. I'm kind of panicking. I worked with another acupuncturist for two years with no baby to show for it." She held her palms out face-up and shook her head. "I'm losing faith in everything, including acupuncture, but I've heard such good things about you, I figured—what do I have to lose?"

I gently convinced her to give it three to four months. This presented a challenge, as it was the dead of winter in a particularly snowy year, and she lived in a neighboring state, Wyoming, over an hour away. She agreed to see me every other week and give it 100 percent.

Kristi had been to the local fertility doctor and tried Metformin, Clomid, Letrozole, and one intrauterine insemination (IUI). An IUI is a fertility treatment that involves injecting sperm inside a woman's uterus to increase the chances of fertilization. Her husband's semen analysis was within the normal range, and tests showed that her eggs were in great shape. She had been diagnosed with polycystic ovary syndrome (PCOS), as her cycles were irregular, coming a little late, at every 32-33 days. We both agreed that this wasn't particularly irregular, so she decided to stop the Metformin.

Metformin lowers blood sugar, as many PCOS patients are insulin resistant. Lowering blood sugar in women with PCOS encourages androgens to correct themselves, which in turn allows for ovulation. While thin women can have insulin resistance, this didn't seem to be the case with Kristi based on her presentation and her clean diet. PCOS presents with a variety of symptoms, including very irregular periods, fluid-filled cysts in the ovaries, and excess levels of androgens (male hormones) causing facial or excess body hair. Women are sometimes incorrectly diagnosed with PCOS if they have only one or two of the defining symptoms, because the real cause of their infertility is unclear. Chinese medicine is effective in correcting imbalances that Western medicine doesn't recognize. My goal was to uncover the real imbalance going on in Kristi.

Kristi had one odd symptom unrelated to her PCOS diagnosis—extremely itchy hives on her lower legs every night starting at 7:00 p.m. I wasn't sure what to make of this, but it was an interesting indication of inflammation. Inflammation is never good for fertility, so it was important to take care of it.

To ease her frustration at doing everything right and still not getting what she wanted, I had her start taking Chinese herbs to take the edge off. She had pain with her cycles, pain with ovulation, and a pulse that indicated she had significant blood stagnation, so I put her on other herbs to help thin her blood. I also recommended that she take maca—Peruvian ginseng—to help balance her hormones.

Kristi had two copies of the MTHFR gene mutation, which was likely interfering with her fertility. Women with this gene mutation don't process folic acid properly, which causes problems for women trying to conceive. I'd surmise that most of my fertility patients carry at least one copy of this mutation. I have two copies myself. It is easily treated by putting the patient on methylated folate instead of folic acid. I recommend that every patient take a top-of-the-line prenatal vitamin that contains L-methylfolate and methylated B12. Sometimes this is all it takes to help them get pregnant, but often, there are more underlying issues that need to be solved, as in Kristi's case.

Taking blood-movers alleviated the pain with her periods, and her brown flow reddened over time. Her ovulations were no longer painful, either. Because her hives were still a problem, I sent her to the functional medicine MD in town, and he suggested that she stop eating gluten, oats, coffee, and dairy products. Given that

Kristi's diet was already so clean, she wasn't happy about more dietary restrictions. However, her hives cleared up almost immediately. After reintroducing some of these foods, she determined that oats were the culprit. She hadn't come for treatment to figure this out, but she was relieved to be rid of this uncomfortable symptom. Morning oatmeal wasn't worth an evening scratch-fest.

The functional medicine doctor also had her take a natural thyroid supplement to shift her thyroid-stimulating hormone (TSH) into the perfect range for conception.

In April, after four months of treatment, Kristi sent me an email to tell me she was pregnant for the first time in her life. I asked her what she thought had done the trick, and she said it was impossible to pinpoint exactly. However, she thought the combination of approaches had made all the difference. I think it was the blending of functional medicine and Chinese medicine, but also a huge dose of her willingness to take all the suggestions the MD and I made.

Kristi wrote this lovely review:

After almost six years of trying to conceive and two years working with another acupuncturist, I decided to see Rachel as a last-ditch effort. After three months with Rachel (and now being 37 years old), we had decided that maybe we should also schedule an appointment with a fertility specialist to get a little more aggressive (much to our chagrin). However, a month later, we canceled our fertility appointment. Why? Because at exactly four months of treatment coupled with the vitamins Rachel recommended, I'm happy to say that I'm finally pregnant! We are still in shock. Thank you so much!

When she was 11 weeks pregnant, Kristi came to see me in a panic. She was frightened by a subchorionic hemorrhage. This is not uncommon in women who have blood stagnation issues.

Fortunately, all was well, and the hemorrhage resolved itself. In December, almost exactly one year after starting treatment with me, she delivered a perfect baby boy. Two years after that, without any treatment, she delivered a brother for her son.

She reflected on the time she thought she'd never have children. "You're a miracle worker, Rachel! You're in the business of making dreams come true."

NEVERTHELESS, SHE PERSISTED

"I'm lopsided," Mary said, chuckling as she answered my intake questions. "Which could be part of the problem."

"What do you mean?" I asked, wondering how to write that in my client notes.

"I have just one fallopian tube. I had my right one removed in 2012 because there was a large cyst attached to it."

We both knew that with only one fallopian tube, her chances of conception were lower than if she had two. I reassured her that I had seen plenty of women conceive with only one tube.

"Acupuncture feels like my last hope," she said with her fingers interlocked in her lap. "Do you think you can help? I have already been to the fertility doctor, and I feel like it's time to try this from a different perspective."

"Let's see what we can do. Acupuncture has been the last resort for many of my patients, and we've had some surprisingly awesome results."

Mary first came to see me in 2015 when she was 36. A healthy, fit woman who biked everywhere, she and her husband grew much of their own food and ate beautiful home-cooked meals. She had a normal BMI and was healthy other than some acne on her forehead and cheeks. She had been pregnant two and a half years earlier, but her pregnancy had ended in miscarriage at 12 weeks.

Before she came to see me, Mary had consulted with the local fertility doctor (reproductive endocrinologist or "RE") who unearthed some issues. In 2014, she had surgery to remove endometriosis and a septum in her uterus. A septate uterus is divided in half by membrane. This divided uterus doesn't supply the necessary blood and nutrients to the developing embryo if it happens to implant onto the septum. Women with this condition are at increased risk of miscarriage until it is corrected with surgery.

After her surgery, and with the RE's help, she had tried four cycles of Clomid (to recruit the eggs), Menopur (to develop even more eggs), and HCG (to force the eggs to ovulate). Two of those cycles were also IUIs, and none were successful. That's when she decided to try fertility acupuncture.

Taking Clomid had heated up Mary internally; she awakened at night with hot flashes. She also had many signs of a methylation disorder (where one doesn't process folic acid properly), including infertility, miscarriage, a septate uterus, blood stagnation (aka endometriosis), and a family history of anxiety, depression, and cancer.

I initially treated her with blood-moving herbs to help thin her blood and treat the underlying cause of the endometriosis. Recurrent yeast infections had plagued her since her endometriosis surgery, so I recommended an herbal douche. It helped, but it wasn't enough, so she took Diflucan to clear it up.

For three months, she came in weekly, and she was pregnant by the Fourth of July! She quickly developed a rash on her chest and achy joints, both symptoms of an immune reaction to the pregnancy. I put her on herbs to decrease inflammation and her overactive immune response. It seemed to help, as her rash and achy joints subsided. Her yeast infection returned, and she suffered from nausea and heartburn.

An ultrasound showed a gestational sac and a yolk sac, but no heart flicker yet. Because it was still early, around six weeks, the RE said to not worry—sometimes that heartbeat doesn't show up for a few more days. Ominously, the ultrasound also showed two fluid pockets and a polyp in her uterus. She began spotting brown blood after the ultrasound. The rash moved to her belly button, and her throat was still sore, both signs that an immune reaction was still happening. She continued the formula to treat her overactive immune system.

The next time I saw her, she slumped in the waiting room and stared blankly at the wall. I approached her, touched her shoulder, and said, "Are you okay?"

Before she sat down in the chair next to mine in my treatment room, she burst into tears.

"What happened?" I asked.

Mary spoke through tears. "The ultrasound technician tried so hard to find a heartbeat. As she moved the wand around inside me, I realized that I was probably going to have another miscarriage." Mary sobbed into her palms.

"It's okay. Take all the time you need," I said.

"The heart never flickered. It didn't have a heartbeat." She peered at her hands and was silent.

"Mary, I hope you know this had nothing to do with you. Many early pregnancies don't make it because of a defect or some other problem. In fact, a quarter of all pregnancies end in miscarriage—it's just that most women miscarry before they even realize that they are pregnant.

"Jump up on the table, and I'll give you a treatment that will help you feel better. And I have herbs to heal your uterus, cool you down, and help you feel better."

She continued to come in weekly, and together, we worked to help her get pregnant again.

During the dilation and curettage (D&C) procedure Mary received after she lost the pregnancy, the RE found a piece of the septum in her uterus that hadn't been completely removed and noted it in her chart. During her first period after the D&C, Mary had the worst cramping she had ever experienced. The RE ran a panel of immune blood tests. He also ran a miscarriage panel and discovered that her beta-2-glycoprotein was slightly elevated, indicating that her body makes antiphospholipid antibodies (APAs).

APAs are a group of immune proteins that the body produces against itself in an autoimmune response to phospholipids in cell walls. APAs increase the risk of excessive blood clotting, which can cause a developing embryo to miscarry. They can also contribute to pre-eclampsia, a condition that raises blood pressure to dangerous levels near the end of pregnancy, threatening the baby's and the mother's life. Treatment of APAs to complete a successful pregnancy is with injectable blood thinners (Lovenox) after a woman first becomes pregnant. It looked like Mary would have to do this the next time she became pregnant.

A hysteroscopy showed a tiny polyp, and indeed, a ridge where the septum had previously been removed. Mary scheduled surgery to remove the ridge. In the meantime, her husband had a double knee replacement. While she waited to have the surgery and get back on the trying-to-conceive (TTC) bandwagon, we continued to clear heat and move blood. She was overheated at night and experiencing cramps with her cycle. I wanted to help her address these symptoms before she tried to conceive again. Mary was still trying to get her yeast infections under control. Yeast infections indicated too much dampness in her system. Hot flashes and acne indicated a heat imbalance.

After thinking about it, Mary opted not to have the surgery after all, and 11 months after starting treatment, and eight months after her D&C, she was pregnant again. She miscarried almost immediately at less than five weeks. The RE recommended putting her on Lovenox and baby aspirin, both blood thinners, to proactively treat the APA syndrome the next time she became pregnant.

She and her husband took three months off from trying to conceive, and the first month they tried again, in July of 2016, she became pregnant! Her doctor immediately put her on Lovenox injections and baby aspirin to prevent her from miscarrying. Her HCG levels rose dramatically— quadrupling—from 33 to 112 to 433, indicating that she could be pregnant with more than one baby.

Mary started to experience autoimmune symptoms again—a sore throat but no rash this time. Her first ultrasound at six weeks and three days showed no heartbeat. Her symptoms had disappeared at six weeks and one day, a likely indication of when she had lost the baby. This was now her third miscarriage since starting acupuncture, and her fourth in total. The RE suggested genetic testing and rescheduling surgery to have the remaining bit of septum removed.

In addition to the surgery, Mary had even more tests. She did a monitored, unmedicated cycle to reveal her estrogen levels at ovulation. She also had an endometrial biopsy to test for uterine infection and tests to determine estrogen and progesterone levels in the second half of her cycle. She continued her acupuncture and herbal treatment. Her blood levels looked normal, and the biopsy showed no infection in her uterus. For the fourth time since starting acupuncture and herbs, she was pregnant! This was 21 months after starting acupuncture treatment and over four years since her first pregnancy which ended in miscarriage. Again, she had cold/virus/autoimmune symptoms, so I put her on herbs to calm her immune system. She injected Lovenox and took baby aspirin. She had all the normal pregnancy symptoms—sore breasts, nausea, and heartburn. Her HCG was extremely high, and her sore throat subsided. At six weeks and one day, an ultrasound showed a heartbeat! She called me with the news and said, "I guess I can grow a baby with a heartbeat." But then she was quiet.

"Are you still there?" I asked, thinking we had lost the connection.

"Yeah, sorry. I just realized I don't want to jinx it!"

During Mary's second ultrasound at eight and a half weeks, the baby looked good. She had no more autoimmune symptoms, so she stopped taking the herbs. At 12 weeks, everything looked great. At 13 weeks, she caught a cold, but it seemed like a real cold this time, not an immune reaction, and it quickly disappeared. The rest of her pregnancy was uneventful, thankfully.

Mary returned to my office at 36 weeks to prepare for labor. Acupuncture before labor relaxes the cervix and pelvic floor to facilitate an easy delivery. Mary switched her blood thinner from Lovenox to heparin to prepare for delivery, as the effects of heparin are easier to reverse quickly if she were to bleed too much during delivery.

Her baby boy was sunny side up, which caused an uncomfortable delivery. But he was healthy at six pounds, four ounces. After delivery, Mary sought treatment with me to improve her milk supply. It was wonderful for Mary to be able to talk about her beautiful baby boy instead of yet another miscarriage or uterine surgery. Normal newborn problems like sleep deprivation and low milk supply were put into perspective after everything she had been through.

When Jake was 13 months old, Mary came to see me, thinking of trying for baby number two. She was 40 and wanted to get going before it was too late. Her Chinese medical pattern was the same as the first time she came in, so I put her on heat-clearing herbs and blood movers to boost her fertility.

At age 40 and three months, she began TTC again. Her husband had to repeat knee replacement surgery. This delayed her ability to try for several months, as his body was under stress from surgery, and he needed to clear the anesthesia from his system. In the meantime, we worked on clearing heat and moving blood again and getting her body in shape for a successful pregnancy.

Nine months after restarting acupuncture, Mary was pregnant again! She immediately went on blood thinners. Unfortunately, the pregnancy didn't last, and she had a fifth miscarriage. Mary was now 41, an age at which, in combination with her autoimmune issue increased her odds of miscarriage.

Nevertheless, she persisted.

A month later, when her husband, Peter, showed up on my table for treatment, I was surprised to see him. He didn't have any apparent issues with sperm, but he was 47 years old, and the couple had decided to give their last try everything they had. Research shows that even after three weeks of treatment, sperm count and quality show statistically significant improvement. Women only release one, sometimes two, eggs every month, whereas men make an average of 40 million to 300 million sperm daily in each ejaculation.

On average, men produce 1,000-1,500 sperm with every heartbeat (!), leading to quality issues. Since cell division happens so fast, there is room for error, such as double-headed or double-tailed sperm or sperm with oddly shaped heads—all funny visuals, like strange sea creatures from the deep. But because men manufacture so many sperm, the potential for positive change with treatment is great and happens quickly.

Men represent just 5 percent of my patients, so Peter was in the top percentile. He was a trooper, as he wasn't a fan of acupuncture. But he loved his wife, and he really wanted another child, so he came in weekly. Peter also quit smoking—no small feat. Smart, though, because smoking cessation dramatically improves sperm health.

Mary came in again weekly, and she seemed emotionally down; perhaps she wondered if treatment was a waste of time.

Four months after she returned, and three months after her husband came in for treatment, she was pregnant again at age

41½! This was her sixth pregnancy during our five years of working together. Thankfully, this one worked, and after a healthy and uneventful pregnancy, she gave birth to another bouncing baby boy! It took Mary and Peter many tests and a lot of doctors' and acupuncture appointments to grow their family, but in the end, they felt their persistence was worth it.

UTERINE ANOMALIES: A "UNICORNUATE" UTERUS?

Uterine anomalies are rare in the general population at around 5 percent, though a bit more frequent in the world of infertility. If a woman has a history of infertility or frequent miscarriage, she should certainly get checked out to see if her uterus is normal.

It's surprising the number of things that can go awry during uterine development when a woman is just a fetus in her mother's womb. Some uteruses are heart shaped. Others are separated by a thin membrane called a septum. In a developing female fetus, the two "horns" of the uterus are supposed to fuse together to make a normally shaped uterus. However, some never fuse and end up having two horns. When only one side develops, a woman will have only one horn!

It is always a surprise to a woman to discover she has a uterine malformation, as it's not something she can see or feel.

DOUBLE TROUBLE

Liza, a quick, funny, and anxious therapist came to see me after trying for about six months to conceive baby number two. She and her husband already had a three-year-old son, and they were ready for another child. Pushing her dark hair behind her ears, she revealed her unique health history during her intake assessment.

"Well, you see, I started having periods when I was nine and a half."

"Wow! That's early," I said. "Most start around twelve."

"No kidding! I was so embarrassed around my friends. I kept it a secret for years! But that's not even the weirdest part."

"Oh?" Now, my curiosity was piqued.

"When I went in for a pelvic exam at sixteen, I learned that I got a two for one deal," Liza said. "Lucky me!"

I had no idea what she was talking about.

"I have not one but two uteruses," she said, smiling.

What? It was the first time I had ever heard of this, but I didn't want her to feel like a medical anomaly, so I maintained my clinician's calm veneer and acted like I knew what she was talking about.

"It's called a didelphic uterus," said Liza.

Of course, when our session finished, I fired up my computer and googled it. I learned that one in 3,000 women have a didelphic uterus. It's usually not discovered until a woman has her first gynecological exam, and even then, it can be missed if there is only one vagina. *Wait, only one vagina?* It's true. Some women have two vaginas in addition to the two uteri, but usually only one is functional.

The uterus of an embryonic girl forms between 9- and 20-weeks' gestation. During this time, the two Müllerian ducts usually fuse into a single uterus. This is where things can go awry. A woman with a didelphic uterus often has two cervixes and two vaginas. Some have only one cervix and one vagina. A typical womb has two fallopian tubes and two ovaries, but in Liza's case, each uterus has one tube and one ovary. In women like Liza, the uteri, cervixes, and vaginas are smaller than they would be if the fusion had happened normally. The cause of fusion failure is unknown. The uteri aren't always the same size, and one or both can be functional. Some women even have two periods a month—one from each uterus. One period a month is enough!

Women with a didelphic uterus have a more challenging time getting pregnant and a higher risk of miscarriage, premature labor, and cervical incompetence. The cervix can open before it should, causing a premature delivery, or in the worst case, a late-term miscarriage. Such patients need to be monitored closely during pregnancy but can still deliver a healthy baby. These women may need a cerclage—a stitch in the cervix—during pregnancy to keep the cervix closed and the baby inside. These babies are often breech and need to be delivered by C-section. It's more complicated but not impossible.

At this point, you may be wondering, "What other uterine anomalies can occur during embryonic development?"

The least serious condition is an arcuate uterus, a mildly heart-shaped uterus. It is not usually implicated in fertility issues, though patients can have an increased risk of endometriosis. Many of my patients have had this diagnosis and delivered healthy, full-term babies.

The next level up, more serious, is a septate uterus or one divided by a septum or membrane. This can precipitate frequent miscarriages but can be corrected by a skilled surgeon. Once a patient's septum is removed, she can usually become and stay pregnant. I frequently see this in the clinic.

The next level up is a bicornuate uterus, where the uterus is divided into two separate horns by a thicker septum. This gives it a pronounced heart shape, as seen on imaging. If the deformity is not too severe, it can be corrected with surgery. The patient must wait at least three months after surgery to conceive. Because the patient has undergone uterine surgery, doctors strongly recommend a C-section at delivery to avoid a uterine rupture.

The final uterine anomaly I'll mention here has my favorite name—the "unicornuate" or one-horned uterus. In this case, only one horn develops during fetal development, though there is often a much smaller functional or nonfunctional horn, giving the uterus a banana shape. This rare condition makes it quite difficult to conceive. There is a greater risk of miscarriage or pre-term delivery, and it sometimes results in an ectopic pregnancy. A woman with a unicornuate uterus needs a cerclage to keep the baby inside, as her uterus is smaller than normal, and the baby can grow too large to remain in utero full term. A unicornuate uterus is the rarest of uterine anomalies—affecting only 1 to 2 percent of women.

I have seen at most five patients with diagnosed unicornuate uteri in 21 years of practice.

I'm always optimistic about women's chances to conceive because I have seen excellent results in the most challenging circumstances. Even with unusual cases such as these, I encourage and help women to try everything in their pursuit of motherhood.

Years earlier at age 25, Liza and her husband began trying for their first child. Because they had been unsuccessful at such a young age, they visited a gynecologist (OB/GYN) after two years of trying. The OB/GYN surgically removed a septum that was dividing her vagina in two, prohibiting sperm from reaching one of her fallopian tubes. Six months later, they conceived their first son. Because of her small uterus, he was born at 31 weeks, but he was healthy.

Liza faithfully came for treatment for four months. During that time, we had many fantastic conversations as I placed needles over her uteri and ovaries, and in her arms and legs. She also faithfully took herbs to eliminate cramps and improve microcirculation in her uterine lining(s). Liza decided to take a break from acupuncture because she thought she might be pregnant again. When she learned she wasn't, she took leave from work to focus on her health and reduce her stress, including taking an antidepressant and going on a much-needed vacation.

Several months after slowing her life down, Liza was pregnant with her second child. Sometimes the body just needs a little R&R. Her doctor put in a cerclage at 12 weeks to keep her cervix tightly closed. She had experienced many issues in her first pregnancy including gestational diabetes, an incompetent cervix, and an irritable uterus. A generally mild condition, an irritable uterus presents as irregular, mini contractions that can be treated with rest, relaxation, proper hydration, caffeine elimination, and keeping the bladder as empty as possible. The bladder sits next to the uterus and puts pressure on it when it is full. However, in a case like Liza's where the uterus is smaller than normal, her irritable uterus needed to be controlled by stronger measures with Western drugs.

Liza's second pregnancy wasn't easy. At 13 weeks, her doctor put her on antibiotics for a week because he suspected an underlying infection causing the uterine irritability. Things such as a bladder infection from intercourse or hot-tub use could have caused it. Despite the antibiotics, she continued to experience discomfort, and at 18 weeks, she reported uterine pressure and sharp twinges around 70 percent of the time. During this time, she learned that her grandmother was dying, adding another layer of stress.

At 22 weeks, Liza was hospitalized due to contractions and took medication to control them. The medicine made her tired but did the trick. Sadly, she lost her grandmother during this time. Her grief was intense, but fortunately her pregnancy progressed.

At 25 weeks, Liza was having up to 12 contractions an hour, which would normally frighten doctors into thinking she was going into labor soon. Her ultrasounds showed that the baby was fine, and it turned out she wasn't about to deliver. Heroically, she was able to keep her second son inside until 32 weeks, one week longer than her first son. Her functional uterus was stretched out after the first pregnancy and could accommodate the second baby a week longer.

A couple of years later, Liza called me and let me know that her third and final son came at 33 weeks—relatively late for her. Her uterus had stretched a little bit more! Unfortunately, each pregnancy had successively more complications, requiring more medical interventions and longer bed rest.

Having beaten the odds three times, Liza knew she was done having children. She had grown three healthy sons, albeit premature, with her unusual uterus. Liza says that despite all the complications and stress that accompanied each pregnancy, she is grateful for each of her sons, and would do it all over again.

AGAINST ALL ODDS

Katrin, an evolutionary biologist and science professor at a nearby university, came to see me in September of 2017 at age 35½, aware that her fertility window was narrowing. Although American, Katrin still had a touch of a Swiss-German accent after living in Switzerland as a post-doc for a couple of years. Petite and fit with long brown hair and blue eyes, she had never been pregnant before. She had been trying to conceive for only one month, but she knew that her markers determining optimal fertility were off, and she wanted to act swiftly to correct them. Her FSH was slightly elevated at around 13 mIU/ml (healthy levels are below 10), and her AMH was a little low at 0.76 ng/ml (optimal levels are above 1). Not the worst, but not outstanding. Nevertheless, I was convinced it was worth a try.

Her menstrual cycles were mostly normal but with mild cramps and some spotting in the luteal phase. Spotting in the second half or luteal phase of a woman's cycle can indicate low levels of progesterone at a time when high levels are needed to continue a pregnancy. Katrin might require progesterone supplementation if her test results showed it to be low. I recommended that she also have her Vitamin D3 and thyroid-stimulating hormone (TSH) levels tested. Her D3 was only 30 nmol/L—within normal limits—but should be closer to 50 nmol/L for optimal fertility. Her TSH was 3.1 mU/L, also within normal limits, but fertility doctors like to see it between 1 and 2 for the best chances of success.

Katrin lived an hour and a half's drive from my clinic, so she came in every other week instead of weekly like most of my clients. After three months of treatment with acupuncture and herbs, she was still spotting in the luteal phase, although her menstrual flow was brighter red, a sign of improved uterine circulation. After she started thyroid medication prescribed by her OB/GYN, her thyroid levels were in a more optimal range.

A month later, she and her partner went to a Colorado fertility clinic for an evaluation. Her partner's semen analysis checked out, but an ultrasound revealed that Katrin had a unicornuate uterus, a rare genetic condition in which only one-half of a female's uterus forms. A unicornuate uterus is smaller than a typical uterus and has only one fallopian tube. This results in a shape often referred to as "a uterus with one horn" or a "single-horned uterus." Thus, the name "unicornuate." A unicornuate uterus occurs in just 0.1 percent of the general population. Katrin considered buying a lottery ticket for a moment, as her odds of winning now seemed about as good as her odds of having this condition.

After learning this critical information, the clinic said Katrin couldn't take fertility drugs because of the risk of becoming pregnant with multiple embryos. Gestating one baby to full term with a unicornuate uterus is difficult or sometimes impossible, and the risk of miscarriage is high. Getting pregnant with more than one baby would be too dangerous for Katrin and her babies. Ever the researcher, Katrin threw herself into learning everything she could about her condition. She didn't have time to waste feeling sorry for herself because of the cards she had been dealt. She wanted a baby!

Five months after starting acupuncture treatment and taking supplemental progesterone, Katrin became pregnant naturally. We were both so excited! The pregnancy progressed normally until, unfortunately, she miscarried at nine weeks due to Trisomy 22, a genetic defect that is incompatible with life. Katrin grieved and took time to recover.

Katrin switched fertility doctors, and the new reproductive endocrinologist monitored her cycle for a luteal phase defect because of the spotting in the second half of her cycle. He also thought he saw an unconnected horn on her unicornuate uterus. A unicornuate uterus often only has one fallopian tube, but hers had the beginnings of a second one. This was an outgrowth where the fallopian tube might have grown, but it was closed. He was concerned that she risked ectopic pregnancy or uterine rupture if she conceived either naturally or by IVF. He recommended surgery to remove the tiny horn.

Katrin was initially hesitant to do the surgery because she didn't want to delay trying to get pregnant. She eventually agreed because the RE was convinced that she needed the surgery. At this point, Katrin had been in acupuncture treatment for a year. Her FSH had risen to 17.4, and her AMH had decreased to 0.46, creating anxiety about her fertility. I prescribed Chinese herbs to improve her egg health and alleviate her night sweats.

The surgery was delayed by a month, but it was finally completed. Her doctor removed the tiny horn and tube and removed some endometriosis he discovered.

While healing, Katrin researched "mini-IVF" in which far less of the IVF medicines are administered, putting less stress on the body. At the time, the relatively new mini-IVF was making news because it showed success in women like Katrin with higher FSH and lower AMH. These women were often turned away from IVF clinics but could have success with a mini-IVF. This process is becoming more popular as it has shown promising results with fewer side effects. Her RE agreed to try it, though he had never done one before. Ever the advocate for herself, Katrin researched REs who had more experience doing mini-IVF and chose a clinic in a neighboring Western state.

Katrin had a decent number of follicles to proceed but soon discovered the clinic was in chaos due to poor management and communication. Just as she was about to start a mini-IVF, they asked, "This is a traditional IVF, right?" She quickly canceled. It had been only four months since her last evaluation, but her AMH was falling again, down to 0.31 from 0.48. She had no time to waste with suboptimal clinics. Katrin switched to a new clinic in California with a stellar reputation. This clinic recommended three egg retrievals three months in a row to bank fertilized embryos for future use. This is a genius method of extracting as many eggs as possible before a woman's eggs get any older.

During her first retrieval, she produced six eggs, two of which were mature. Neither was genetically normal. For her second egg retrieval, the clinic used minimal drugs and retrieved three eggs, one of which fertilized and was frozen, as it was genetically normal. Her third retrieval produced 11 good eggs, 6 of which fertilized. Three were genetically normal, and they were frozen. So, in total, she had four healthy embryos. After genetic testing, it was determined that they were two boys and two girls.

As a scientist and a motivated mother-to-be, Katrin was a tireless advocate for herself. She wasn't interested in wasting a single embryo to miscarriage, and since blood tests had revealed some issues with her immune system, she found a reproductive immunologist in Chicago who could help her manage potential immunological issues. With four extremely valuable, hard-won embryos and an AMH of only 0.3, she couldn't afford to waste a single embryo or undergo any more retrievals, so she carefully followed the immunologist's suggestions on how best to proceed.

At this point, I was more of a cheerleader for Katrin than anything else, but optimism and encouragement always help. I learned a lot about reproductive immunology and treating immune issues in fertility during this process.

Katrin had borderline-elevated tumor necrosis factor (TNF), which is great for fighting off cancer but not so great for a developing embryo. With elevated TNF, her body would have fought off an embryo in her uterus, so her immunologist recommended measures including taking prednisone and tacrolimus to calm her over-reactive immune system. The immunologist also found that Katrin had a genotype linked with various pregnancy complications, including poor glucose metabolism and blood-clotting disorders. To correct for these, Katrin would need to start Metformin to balance glucose metabolism and inject the blood thinner Lovenox during her pregnancy. Still, Katrin did not feel defeated—she was happy to do anything to make her pregnancy stick.

Before her embryo transfer, Katrin also had an endometrial receptivity test so her doctor could pinpoint the date and time of the transfer to perfectly match when her uterus would be most receptive to an embryo. Once her test results came back, Katrin resumed pre-implantation acupuncture with me to help thicken her lining and increase blood flow to her uterus.

Before her transfer, Katrin started Lovenox, Metformin, and immune-suppressing drugs. She researched intravenous immunoglobulin (IVIg) therapy to prevent pregnancy loss, and since her natural killer (NK) cell activity was elevated, she decided to do one course of treatment. IVIg therapy significantly increases live birth rates when administered before conception in patients with recurrent pregnancy loss.

Cupping therapy has also been shown to reduce NK cell activity, so we did that at her next treatment. Cupping is an ancient Chinese medical practice of placing glass or plastic cups on the body after removing the air from them either with fire (quickly, so the glass doesn't get hot) or with a suction mechanism. They taught us "fire cupping" in acupuncture school, which is dramatic and makes for great TV, but there is a risk of burning the patient, so I use boring old suction cups.

Finally, at 38 years old, two years and three months after starting acupuncture, and after advocating for herself like no doctor ever had, a single female embryo was transferred to Katrin's primed, unicornuate uterus. It didn't work. That was in early October 2019. She again prepared for a transfer in November but had to cancel at the last minute because she started bleeding and her progesterone was very low.

Finally, the stars aligned for another transfer in early December, and, to everyone's delight, it worked! Again, Katrin chose a female embryo because she anticipated a premature birth due to her small uterus. Female preemies tend to fare better than males. She wanted to give her hard-won embryo the best chance of survival.

Katrin sent me an update when she was 29 weeks pregnant. Between 23 and 25 weeks, she had been concerned about delivering early due to a shortened cervix, but that corrected itself, and the pregnancy continued. The baby was measuring small and had fallen from the 50thpercentile to the 25th, but Katrin wasn't too concerned as the 25th percentile is still fine.

Katrin wrote again at 35 weeks to report that the baby's size had fallen from the 20th percentile to below 3 percent, a sign that she wasn't growing well anymore, so the OB planned to deliver her baby by C-section at 37 weeks. The baby was breech, most likely because Katrin's uterus was too small for her to turn around in. It was cramped in there! A C-section would be the least stressful birth option for her tiny baby.

Interestingly, I wrote this story on July 30, which turned out to be Katrin's delivery date. Her story wanted to be born at the same time as her baby.

In an email, Katrin wrote: *All went great, and we sure love this tiny peanut already! 4lbs 11oz, and we are still working on a name :) She exceeded the NICU weight cutoff by 126g and has been with us the whole time. She is doing so well! Thank you for all your support on the long road to this point!*

Overcome with joy for Katrin, her husband, and her tiny baby, I once again realized that I have the best job ever.

IVF:
TEST TUBE BABIES

In July of 1978, the first "test tube" baby, Louise Brown, was born in England. Her mother, Lesley Brown, suffered from infertility due to blocked fallopian tubes. At one time, a woman like her with severe blockages or a complete lack of fallopian tubes would never have been able to carry her own child, but thanks to innovations in reproductive technology, they now can. Men with almost no sperm in their ejaculate or very compromised sperm can father their own children using IVF with intracytoplasmic sperm injection (ICSI). Sperm cells can sometimes be extracted from the testicles, and then injected into waiting eggs. A true miracle of science!

One might argue that IVF is overused, since it is sometimes a first resort after a period of infertility, but for couples with unexplained infertility or reproductive obstacles they can't overcome, it is a huge blessing.

THE GIFT OF LIFE

The first thing that struck me about Emily was her beauty. Her long, tightly curled hair was offset by her ice-blue eyes. The second thing was the acne dotting her chin and cheeks. While common in adolescence, acne is unusual in people of Emily's age—27. Most, upon seeing Emily's acne would think, "dermatologist." Few would think, "acupuncturist." But her acne held a clue to the words written on her paperwork—*cannot conceive*. In Chinese face reading, the chin represents the uterus and ovaries, and the cheeks represent the intestines. Chin and cheek acne indicate blood stagnation in the lower *jiao*—the part of the body that houses the uterus, ovaries, and intestines.

Emily had been trying to conceive for 20 months, but none of the commonly run fertility tests pointed to infertility; her bloodwork was normal, and her HSG showed that her tubes were open. She was being treated by our local, beloved RE. She reported severe pain with ovulation, which, like her acne, was a sign of blood stagnation. Her cycles were sometimes short, just 24-27 days, and intensely painful on days one and two, including pain radiating through her intestines and rectum; both symptoms can indicate endometriosis. Her breasts were tender before her cycle, and she suffered from premenstrual insomnia. All her symptoms improved with exercise.

I started Emily on herbs to treat blood stagnation, which caused her period symptoms to intensify. In fact, she said they were the worst she had ever experienced. I honestly don't know why she came back to see me. I might have run the other way if that had happened to me! But over the months of treatment, her ovulation pain disappeared, her sleep improved, and her cramps mostly resolved.

Two months after starting treatment, her 27-year-old husband was diagnosed with lupus. They had been experiencing infertility for almost two years, and on top of everything, Emily had lost both of her grandfathers within six weeks of one another. Her husband's diagnosis felt like salt in the wound. But they hoped that perhaps lupus was the reason for their infertility—that they had finally stumbled upon the answer.

Unfortunately, the rheumatologist told them lupus doesn't affect fertility at all. They were thankful that there was nothing "wrong" with them, but it was incredibly frustrating to not know the root cause of their infertility. How would they find a solution?

The next year was a blur. Dave was desperately sick. It was a major distraction to their infertility, but it certainly solved the answer to, *if you forget about getting pregnant, that's when it happens*. Having a baby was the last thing on their minds. They were still "trying" in that they weren't using birth control, but Emily was so busy keeping her husband healthy that she lost track of her cycles. One night after they had gone to the ER, they were driving home at 3:00 a.m. and Emily pulled over because Dave needed to vomit from his prescribed pain medicine.

After the waves of nausea passed, he took Emily's hand and said, "Aren't you so glad we aren't taking care of a toddler right now?"

She nodded and said, "Always a silver lining—right?"

In that moment, they were grateful but also a bit regretful. They wished Dave didn't have lupus and that they actually did have a toddler. They are firm believers that everything happens for a reason, so in that moment, they were grateful that they didn't also have a toddler to raise.

Dave was seriously ill for about a year. He received steroid infusions through a port in his arm over a five-day course, and that turned things around. He is now maintained on a very basic medication. He has little flareups here and there, but nothing to the extent of that first year.

Six months into Emily's treatment, the RE ordered a laparoscopy—a surgical procedure in which a fiber-optic instrument is inserted through the patient's abdominal wall to view the uterus and ovaries. She also had a colonoscopy, which showed that her large intestine was healthy. Not surprisingly, she had extensive endometriosis in her uterus and on her intestines, which the RE removed. Initially, after surgery, she was thrilled to be in no pain. However, nine days later, she had horrible cramping and the heaviest period she had experienced since high school.

The next two cycles after her laparoscopy were much less painful, with no pain in her intestines or rectum, which was a huge relief! Her cycles shortened to 25 days, but her progesterone was in the normal range when measured, so we knew low progesterone wasn't the culprit. She was put on progesterone anyway to lengthen her cycles, and it made her feel good. As a bonus, it also prevented premenstrual spotting. These signs indicated that she was estrogen-dominant (as is often the case with endometriosis) because the increased progesterone helped alleviate her symptoms.

A year and a half into treatment, an ultrasound revealed that she had a large cyst requiring surgery. Emily couldn't get a break! The surgeon removed a follicular cyst that had calcified into a tumor. Thankfully, it was benign.

After recovering from surgery, she was back on the TTC wagon. By this time, I had learned about the MTHFR gene mutation—a mutation that can interfere with fertility. Signs that one may have it include symptoms of blood stagnation, including bad cramps and a family history of heart attack or stroke. Other, more subtle signs are frequent miscarriages and stubborn infertility. To treat the issues that go along with the MTHFR gene mutation, I put her on a prenatal vitamin that contained folate instead of folic acid. Her skin cleared up quickly, including the acne on her back. While these were welcome changes, Emily was still not pregnant.

Frustrated by no results in three years, she asked her RE to step things up, and he prescribed Clomid. She took it for three months, which only resulted in two cysts. Fortunately, they went away naturally.

I hadn't seen Emily for a year when she returned, and she was almost 31. Pain with her cycles flared up again, which indicated that the endometriosis had likely returned. The RE prescribed Letrozole and Menopur, which produced multiple follicles each time, yet she was still not getting pregnant.

Emily had started acupuncture treatment four years earlier and had been trying for a baby for six. She was now 32 years old. She took a few months off to pray and surround herself with people in her church who loved her. I felt helpless; I had nothing more to offer except love and support.

Eight months later, she came in for treatment. As she lay on the treatment table, she said, "So, you know I can't afford IVF—right?"

"Yes, I'm so sorry." I again felt helpless in the face of her predicament. I so desperately wanted Emily to get a break.

"Well, you're not going to believe what happened," she said, peering into my eyes.

"What?" *Is she pregnant?*

"My husband and I received a gift from a church member."

"Oh?" I wondered what the gift could be.

"We received eighteen thousand dollars for IVF!"

"What?! That's incredible!"

"I know." She glanced up at me, her eyes filled with tears. "It's truly the gift of life!"

My eyes teared up in response, and soon, we were both crying.

"Who gave you the gift?" I asked.

"We don't know. The church member wishes to remain anonymous."

"Wow. I'm blown away by such an act of kindness in our community."

"I know. It's a miracle. Our prayers worked."

Her testing showed that her FSH and AMH were perfect, which made sense because she was still young. During her IVF cycle, she produced 16 eggs, 9 of which fertilized. Six were A+ grade, and three were A's. Things were truly looking up for Emily.

Studies show that for patients who receive acupuncture treatment immediately before and after a "fresh" or day three in vitro procedure, 42.5 percent of the patients in the acupuncture group became pregnant, whereas the pregnancy rate was only 26.3 percent in the control or non-acupuncture group. Emily wanted to do everything to make this work.

On the day of Emily's transfer, I woke up before sunrise and drove to work in the ink-black of the early morning. Emily and I met at 5:45 a.m., so that I could treat her before the transfer. I wouldn't have missed it for the world. She had been my patient for almost five years. I'd have woken at 3:00 a.m. to help her!

As the two microscopic embryos flowed through the catheter into her uterus, I went for a trail run with the rising sun. While Emily rested in the fertility clinic after her embryo transfer, I went back to work and waited for her to come to my office for her post-transfer treatment. Everything had gone perfectly.

During the two-week wait to learn if she was pregnant or not, she had cramping so intense that it felt like a bad period was starting. Cramping during this time is often a sign that an embryo is implanting in the uterus, but this cramping was more intense than many other patients report. In addition, Emily's backside was sore from the progesterone shots she injected into her gluteus muscle every day.

Two weeks after her transfer, she had a positive pregnancy test. Her first ever. She couldn't believe it! Her HCG more than doubled every 48 hours from 90 to 255 and finally to 766 when they stopped testing it. *Could it be twins?*

As it turned out, she wasn't carrying twins, but she had a healthy pregnancy and gave birth to a perfect baby girl, Evelyn. I was mesmerized by her sparkly ice-blue eyes, blonde curls, and darling little face. She is the most beautiful little girl I have ever seen, other than my own daughter, of course. She is a cherished baby, and so precious.

Six and a half years after her very first appointment with me, and two years to the day of the egg retrieval that created the little embryos, Emily returned to prepare for her second embryo transfer, this time a frozen one. The transfer of her daughter's frozen fraternal twin went perfectly.

A year later, I ran into Emily and her gorgeous new baby girl Violet, at the store. I admired the new baby and she caught me up, telling me all about her life now, juggling work, a toddler, and a baby. Running into clients, seeing their pregnant bellies or darling babies and learning the rest of the story are the cherry on top of a most fulfilling job.

Emily said, "Although it didn't feel like it in the moment, looking back I know that Dave's illness made our faith stronger. And our marriage is stronger as well. Every step we took to have our babies helped us appreciate them in a different way. Not a better way than those who can conceive easily, but just a different way. I often still can't believe they're here. There are so many surreal moments when I hear their giggles, or I hear them cry out for Daddy, it takes my breath away. All I can say is, 'Thank you, Jesus. Thank you for letting me be a mama.'"

RUNNING LOW ON EGGS:
LOW ANTI-MÜLLERIAN HORMONE

Anti-Müllerian hormone (AMH) is a measure of the approximate number of eggs left in a woman's ovaries. It doesn't measure quality, but rather the number of eggs remaining. This measurement doesn't always correspond with a woman's age. Unfortunately, young women can be diagnosed with low AMH levels in a condition called premature ovarian failure (POF).

Low AMH (below one) means that a woman's fertility window is closing; it's not the end yet, as a few eggs may remain. Time is of the essence, and treatment should be as soon as possible, whether with a Western or Eastern fertility clinic or, in the best-case scenario, both.

PAST THE EXPIRATION DATE

Xiaomin, a 38-year-old software engineer, came to see me, nervous because her biological clock was ticking. She said it was deafening.

One of the best parts of my job is getting to know my patients. I ask them all kinds of questions because I love hearing their personal stories. Things like *Where did you grow up? What does your husband or partner do? What did you do this weekend?* I find people to be endlessly fascinating.

Xiaomin was all business, so it took time to draw her out, but eventually I made some headway. She already had one child, a 6½-month-old son, and she wanted a sibling for her baby boy. She came to see me with low expectations but with the hope that I could work some magic.

She was seeing an RE in Denver to be evaluated for IVF. But her numbers didn't look good. In fact, they were in a range that would prompt most IVF clinics to turn her away. Her follicle-stimulating hormone (FSH), which measures the health and approximate age of the egg, was 17 IU/ml. The ideal FSH level for IVF is below 10 IU/ml. Her AMH, which measures the quantity of eggs left in the ovaries, was 0.15 ng/ml. Most clinics prefer that AMH is between 1 and 3ng/ml. The number of resting ovarian follicles on day three of a woman's cycle gives the IVF clinic an idea of how well a patient will respond to stimulation medications. An ideal resting follicle count is between 15 and 20. She had only two resting follicles as seen on an ultrasound. Most IVF clinics won't consider doing an IVF when a patient has numbers like hers. Bottom line, things were not looking good, and we had plenty of work to do.

Xiaomin also had endometriosis which caused painful periods, so painful, in fact, that she'd down painkillers just to make it through the day. While we were waiting to see if she could improve her situation with acupuncture to be considered for IVF, I put her on blood-moving herbs to get rid of cramps. These herbs break up blood clots, called "blood stagnation" in Chinese medicine, that cause pain during menstruation. Picture a garden: if a gardener plants seeds in clumpy soil, they are less likely to grow, or to grow well. Blood-moving Chinese herbs "aerate" the soil, making a healthy bed in which the seeds can implant. She reported only a little pain during her next menstrual cycle, and, for the first time, she didn't need painkillers.

Xiaomin wanted to do everything to make her IVF dream happen, so she saw me for treatments twice a week. To boost the health of her eggs, I used points over her sacrum to increase blood flow to her eggs and uterus. She continued this for three months and took the blood-moving herbs I prescribed. She reported less pain, a brighter red flow, and healthier flow with each period. Her uterus "garden" was getting healthier and more receptive to an embryo.

Four months after she started acupuncture treatments, Xiaomin's levels were tested again. Her FSH decreased from 17 to 14, her AMH increased from 0.15 to 0.4, and her ultrasound showed she had five resting follicles, up from two. Her numbers were looking promising but weren't quite there yet.

She was approved for IVF, and to be honest, I was surprised the clinic made this decision. Even though her numbers had improved, they were still not optimal. The clinic must have felt like she would succeed if they were willing to put her through an IVF procedure. Nonetheless, I was there to support my patient no matter what. I remained cautiously optimistic.

Xiaomin started IVF medications five months after starting acupuncture. She continued to see me twice a week. Most people come in twice a week for the four weeks leading up to the embryo transfer, but Xiaomin had been coming in twice a week for four months.

She produced five mature eggs, four of which fertilized. This was truly an amazing result, considering that only half of the retrieved eggs fertilize in most IVFs. The RE transferred one embryo into her uterus, which successfully burrowed in and implanted.

Xiaomin delivered a healthy baby boy in the nick of time, just before her biological clock stopped ticking. She was relieved she had decided to pair Eastern and Western medicine to enhance her fertility and make her dream of expanding her family possible. I'm certain her frequent acupuncture treatments, plus herbs and her intense commitment, made all the difference.

ADVANCED MATERNAL AGE: TOO OLD TO HAVE CHILDREN?

If you're over the age of 35, your pregnancy may be considered high risk due to "advanced maternal age." What woman wants to hear she is of advanced maternal age. How insulting!

This simply means these women are more likely than younger women to have certain conditions and complications that may put them and their baby at risk. It doesn't always mean the end of the fertility road, as evidenced by these stories. Egg quality has to do with a variety of factors, including genetics, environment, and diet.

Staying up all night with your baby may be easier when you are in your twenties and early thirties; however, many older mothers can still experience this quality nighttime with their babies.

SPERM HATS AND EGGS ON ICE

"So, I know I'm starting late, but the stars didn't align for me to have kids until now. My husband and I have been trying for a year with no luck," said Sara, a new 40-year-old patient.

"The good news for you is that things have changed so much. Women have children well into their forties."

"I don't know why I assume it's my fault. Maybe my husband's swimmers can't make it across the channel."

We both chuckled.

"Exactly!" I said.

"Well, he certainly didn't have trouble in his previous marriage. He has five children. But now he's fifty-six."

After three months of acupuncture and herbs to improve her cycles, it was clear that Sara and Ben needed to pursue fertility treatments. Sara's biological clock was tick, tick, ticking away. Her eggs were screaming, *use us or lose us!*

The couple consulted with one of the best IVF clinics in the country.

"So, I was right," said Sara, during a treatment. "My numbers are good for IVF. Ben's sperm are the culprit!"

"A-ha!" I said. "You called it."

"We learned that ninety-one percent of Ben's sperm have anti-sperm antibodies attached to them. I'm not sure what this means, but the doc said it was from Ben's vasectomy, which he had years ago. Then, of course, he had it reversed."

"Think of anti-sperm antibodies like this—imagine a sperm wearing a little hat."

"Okay, I'm picturing a fedora."

We chuckled, imagining fashionable hat-wearing spermatozoa.

"So, an antibody is a hat that the man's body has attached to the sperm to identify it as an invader."

"Why does that happen?"

"If sperm comes into contact with a man's blood, such as during a vasectomy or an injury to the testicles, it sets off an immune response that identifies the sperm as a foreign invader. A man can live with antibody-wearing sperm. However, it's often, but not always, impossible for a sperm with an antibody attached to its head to penetrate an egg. Sperm carry a tiny package of enzymes on their heads called an acrosome. When this attaches to the egg, it breaks down the egg's outer membrane. This is how the sperm gets its DNA into an egg. If a sperm has an antibody hat, the enzymes can't break down the outer layer."

"That makes sense."

"Antibodies can also attach to the sperm's midpiece or tail. In this case, with the presence of antibodies, the sperm are more likely to clump together, making it difficult for them to reach an egg. It is not impossible to get pregnant in the presence of anti-sperm antibodies, but it is quite difficult.

"I had a patient whose two kids were conceived via IVF with intra-cytoplasmic sperm injection or ICSI, where the sperm is injected directly into the egg by an embryologist. Because of her husband's vasectomy, his anti-sperm antibodies interfered. When I later ran into her at the park, she was pregnant again. She told me, remarkably, they conceived baby number three the old-fashioned way. One determined sperm made it through!

"The bottom line is, sometimes the only way for a woman to get pregnant is to undergo IVF with ICSI."

"Hmm… Interesting. We might have to go with ICSI. So many new acronyms to learn."

Sara and Ben chose this approach.

Two months later, the clinic retrieved ten eggs from Sara (not bad for a 40-year-old), seven of which were mature, and six of which fertilized. Unfortunately, only one made it to the blastocyst stage, which is when it was frozen. The clinic sent the blastocyst to Chicago for pre-implantation genetic screening to ensure it had the normal number of chromosomes.

Sara's retrieval triggered severe digestive issues, including shortness of breath, tightness in her throat, and a feeling that she needed to burp but could not. Her doctor ordered chest X-rays and blood tests to rule out a pulmonary embolism. Everything looked normal, so she had an upper endoscopy, and her GI doctor diagnosed her with celiac disease. The clinic delayed the embryo transfer so Sara could recover. Active celiac disease increases the risk of miscarriage and other issues if the gut hasn't recuperated.

While she recovered, the couple decided to harvest more eggs in case the transfer of their only embryo failed. It is a great idea in older women to harvest as many eggs as possible to fertilize for transfer later. That way, each embryo is from the youngest eggs available at the time of retrieval. After age 40, a woman's egg quality takes a nosedive. Keeping some embryos on ice lowers the pressure to have another baby immediately after the first one. Also, it might not always be possible to have another child with the older eggs, so it's good to have an insurance policy.

For three retrieval cycles over nine months, Sara's eggs were retrieved and fertilized—seven embryos the first cycle, one the second cycle, and one the third cycle. None was genetically normal. This left only the one previously frozen embryo to transfer. They transferred it five months after her last retrieval. And they waited. And waited.

And it worked! At long last, Sara was pregnant at 42.

Her clinic ran genetic tests, which showed some mosaicism, a condition in which cells within the same person have a different genetic makeup. Sara, Ben, and the doctors were nervous about this. But it was later determined to have come only from the placenta, not the baby. Baby Otis was born healthy, if not itchy and a bit allergic, just like his mama.

Sara and I stayed in touch. Three years later, I noticed she was on my schedule.

When she came in, she was very pregnant.

"Congratulations, Sara! How far along are you?"

"Thirty-eight weeks. You're not going to believe this, but at forty-six, this one was au naturel! We thought the door was closed, and *voilà*!"

"How did this happen?"

"Apparently, one hatless sperm made it to one of my eggs of advanced maternal age!"

The sneaky sperm that created her baby boy, Shai, had other plans.

EAST MEETS WEST IN FERTILITY TREATMENT

Meeting Johanna felt like a soothing breath of fresh air. It was a delight to work with her. She was smart, forthcoming, a successful pilot, yet humble. Johanna was single, and at 41, she was worried that her fertility window was closing. She didn't want to miss out on having a baby.

At the direction of her OB/GYN, she had tried IUI with Clomid for six months. An IUI fertility treatment involves injecting sperm inside a woman's uterus to increase the chances of fertilization. She had no results, just unpleasant symptoms, including insomnia, bloating, and hot flashes.

Clomid works well for women who tend to run cold and who ovulate later in their cycles. According to Chinese medicine, Clomid is hot in nature, so if a woman is perimenopausal and experiencing heat sensations, such as night sweats, Clomid often exacerbates symptoms. Clomid acts as an estrogen blocker in the hypothalamus, pituitary, ovaries, and female organs. Less estrogen results in increased release of the hormones FSH and LH, which causes the growth of more ovarian follicles, but it also thins the uterine lining, and causes increased heat in women whose bodies are already hot.

Chinese medicine considers the body to be a microclimate. When I hear the word "microclimate," I envision a geodesic dome that houses people or plants. For an embryo to be happy, it can't be too hot, cold, wet, or dry in a woman's "microclimate." Clomid in a woman like Johanna, who is already warm, would make her microclimate way too hot—like a desert in the summer.

Ovulation occurs about six to seven days after starting Clomid. Women take it starting days three to five of their cycle, depending on their doctor's recommendation.

Johanna had her sixth IUI with her OB the day after her first acupuncture treatment. I chose points to balance her hormones, cool her down, and move her liver Qi (energy), since she reported grumpiness and more extreme premenstrual syndrome (PMS) symptoms with increased Clomid. She immediately felt cooler and was no longer waking up sweaty. I also prescribed herbs that she could take at home to continue to move her Qi and cool her down.

Unfortunately, the IUI didn't work, so she left her OB and sought care from an RE. He evaluated her case and prescribed Letrozole, Menopur, and a human chorionic gonadotropin (HCG) trigger shot to make sure that ovulation occurred. Letrozole is much gentler on the body than Clomid in terms of side effects, especially if a woman has internal heat or is blood deficient (i.e., low estrogen). Letrozole's original purpose was to treat breast cancer. When used at the right time in the menstrual cycle, Letrozole promotes ovulation by inhibiting the enzyme aromatase, and suppressing estrogen production. Slightly different from how Clomid works, but different enough to cause fewer side effects.

Between the cooling herbs and the Letrozole, Johanna felt much better during her cycles. Hers is a great example of the effectiveness of working with both Eastern and Western fertility specialists from the outset. Eastern and Western modalities offer powerful options, but they each have their limitations. I can't look inside a uterus and see if there is a blockage preventing pregnancy, like Western medicine can. Western medicine can't see the tiny energetic imbalances preventing pregnancy in a patient's Qi, which is easily corrected by Chinese medicine. When used together, they complement each other, filling the gaps that the other can't.

Johanna became pregnant two months before her 42nd birthday—five months after starting acupuncture and herbs, and in her first month of treatment with an RE. Johanna was lucky to avoid morning sickness, but she experienced hip pain and headaches. She continued treatment with me for relief from her pregnancy symptoms. Johanna delivered a gorgeous baby boy at 40 weeks, much to everyone's delight.

ANCIENT CHINESE MEDICINE SECRET

At 41, Amber came to see me, discouraged about her dream to have a third child and worn out from trying. In the 15 months before she came in for treatment, she had endured first-trimester miscarriages at six, nine, seven and five weeks. She already had two healthy boys, aged six and three, so we knew she was able to get pregnant and carry a healthy baby to term. She had explored the possibility of low progesterone levels, which she thought could be causing the early miscarriages, but her progesterone level during her last pregnancy was 24 ng/ml, which is excellent. Normal levels average 12-20 ng/ml, so that didn't seem to be the problem. Her periods were very light, indicating that she may not have enough uterine lining for an embryo to attach to.

She adhered to a mostly vegan diet but did eat an occasional egg. She worried about her low body weight, so I suggested that she add humanely raised meat if she could tolerate it. Despite her commitment to veganism, she was open to my recommendation, given that she really wanted another child. She was already supplementing her vegan diet with cod liver oil and vitamin B-12, which can be hard to get in a vegan diet.

Amber lived four hours away in the mountains, so a weekly in-person appointment wasn't realistic, especially with young kids. We worked together over the phone and via email. I sent her Chinese herbs customized just for her.

Things weren't moving as quickly as we had hoped, so she agreed to come in for weekly acupuncture sessions for one month, then once a month after that. She added bison to her diet, which is rich in iron, and excellent for building blood as well.

During one of our sessions, Amber revealed that she still had the placenta from one of her sons' pregnancies in the deep freezer. She was planning to plant it under a tree, as some indigenous cultures do, including Native Americans and the Maori of New Zealand. In these cultures, placenta burial symbolizes the baby's link to the earth. In addition, planting a small tree that was "born" in the same year as your child is a lovely way to mark your child's growth.

In TCM, the placenta has been used for hundreds of years as a supplement for patients who are deficient in *jing* and blood. *Jing* is the measure of one's overall strength and vitality. Blood in TCM is more than just the fluid that runs through your veins and flows during menstruation. Blood is used by all the organ systems. Blood deficiency is characterized by pallor, fatigue, dizziness, poor memory and concentration, dry skin and hair, brittle nails, and a light menstrual flow. It is interesting to note how these symptoms correlate to symptoms of dietary iron deficiency, which can happen on a vegetarian diet even if one is as careful as Amber.

It is certainly not my intention to offend vegetarians and vegans by recommending meat consumption. But it's important to note that TCM recommends everything in moderation, including meat. To help Amber get pregnant, she needed to build up her blood and *jing*, and eating meat was the quickest way to do that.

Jing can be compared to the genetic endowment one receives from their parents. Women who are *jing* deficient often feel cold and weak, have issues with their teeth and bones, and with their fertility. As we age, our *jing* reserves decline, and do so more rapidly if we don't stay healthy and take good care of ourselves. Some women are born with low stores of *jing*, but this wasn't the case with Amber. She easily had two children into her late thirties.

Because of Amber's thin uterine lining at the age of 42 and the effects of being a longtime vegan, I suggested that she consume her placenta. Before you get too grossed out, you should know that placentas are an amazing source of nutrition, especially for someone like Amber who was blood deficient. At least it would be her own child's placenta, and not that of an anonymous donor—right?

Placentophagy advocates refer to the *Compendium of Materia Medica*, a comprehensive medical text of TCM from the sixteenth century, as evidence of the long history of postpartum practice and the placenta's medicinal properties. *Zi He Che*, the Chinese term for dried human placenta, has historically been used for treating various ailments, including fatigue and postpartum anxiety and depression. There is some debate in the Western world about the safety and efficacy of consuming placenta, as it filters out toxins before they reach the baby. Selenium, cadmium, mercury, and lead, as well as bacteria have been identified in post-term placental tissues.[1] I don't recommend it to everyone, just those who

---

1. Placentophagy: Therapeutic Miracle or Myth? Cynthia W. Coyle, Ph.D., M.S.,1 Kathryn E. Hulse, Ph.D.,2 Katherine L. Wisner, M.D., M.S.,1 Kara E. Driscoll, M.D.,1 and Crystal T. Clark, M.D., M.Sc.1

are quite deficient. Please consult with an acupuncturist before doing this.

I shared with Amber that I had consumed my placenta after my daughter's birth. Initially, I resisted the idea because it sounded gross, but I knew from my education how valuable it was. My acupuncturist, Kristie, recommended I do so, as my children were only 18 months apart, and I hadn't had much time to recover from the first pregnancy. The thought of stir-frying it sounded revolting, like an even more disgusting version of liver and onions. She assured me that there was no stir-frying involved! She was so insistent that I do it, that she offered to process my placenta for me. I wasn't sure what she meant by processing it. *Freeze-dried placenta? Placenta jerky?*

My husband and I told our midwife of our plans, and since the hospital wasn't open minded about releasing placentas to patients, she had a plan. During my daughter's delivery, our midwife quickly handed the placenta in a bucket to Scott. He sneaked the contraband out of the hospital and into the back of his SUV. My daughter was born on a winter's night, which worked to our advantage. The placenta sat in the SUV overnight and was frozen by morning. The next day, Scott drove it to Kristie who washed it and dehydrated it in her oven while her dogs, intoxicated by the smell, whined and stared at the oven, hoping the treat was for them.

She then ground it into a powder and put it into capsules for me to take, three pills two times a day. I have never felt better than when I was consuming those pills! They were such a tonic to my system, I felt like I was running on rocket fuel. Zoom!

When I finished with the pills, I was sorry they were gone. They made me feel amazing. I was infused with energy and was much less anxious than I had been during the postpartum period with my son. I wanted more but wasn't willing to consume anyone else's placenta, even if it was in capsules. The recovery from my second delivery was relatively easy, and I had enough energy to manage a baby and a 19-month-old toddler.

Upon hearing my anecdote and understanding that it would really help her, Amber was open to the idea, especially since she hadn't buried it yet. I told her there were many options for consuming the placenta, including putting fresh placenta in a smoothie, like one of my patients had tried. Amber said that a placenta smoothie sounded awful. So, she opted for having it processed by a midwife into capsules, which she took daily. Her cycle quickly became redder and heavier.

After 13 months of meeting with me weekly and then monthly, five months after including meat in her diet, and four months after consuming her placenta, Amber became pregnant with a baby girl! She was 43. Amber had an easy, full-term pregnancy, and Jade is now a healthy seven-year-old who adores her two older brothers.

UNEXPLAINED FERTILITY: UNSOLVED FERTILITY MYSTERIES

Sometimes when a woman can't get pregnant, none of the tests her doctor runs reveal an obvious problem. Everything looks normal. So, while the Western doctor is scratching his or her head about unexplained infertility, it's time for other approaches. An imbalance preventing pregnancy isn't always visible to the Western medical eye. This is where fertility acupuncture, supplements, and Chinese herbs really shine. A fertility acupuncturist asks diagnostic questions, feels the patient's pulse, and looks at her tongue to identify the underlying imbalance. The patient is then prescribed herbs, supplements, and a course of acupuncture to rebalance the system.

If a woman's tubes are open, her uterus is healthy, and her husband's sperm is healthy and plentiful, acupuncture and herbs can usually fix the imbalance in three to six months. Acupuncture improves circulation of blood and Qi to the ovaries and uterus, thereby improving outcomes. When blood flow to the uterus is constricted, usually due to a "fight or flight" response, it can be difficult to conceive. Acupuncture relaxes and opens the blood vessels, restoring fertility.

SISTER SECRETS

A client named Anna first came to see me in early September of 2005. At 37, she was a stepmother to two darling girls, but she wanted a biological child before her biological clock stopped ticking. Anna had been trying to get pregnant for several months with no success. After hearing about me through a colleague, she set up an appointment.

Anna told me about her fertility issues, and about her life. As a therapist, she experienced a fair bit of stress and struggled with insomnia and anxiety. She reported being spread thinly between work and home life.

During her evaluation by the fertility doctor, she learned that she had endometriosis, an overgrowth of uterine tissue outside the uterus, which can cause pain and infertility. She had two laparoscopies—outpatient surgeries—to remove endometriosis from her abdominal organs to alleviate pain from her cycles and improve her chances of conception.

Anna told her sister about me, and a week later, Elsa came with her husband to see me for fertility issues. As I greeted Elsa and Rick in the lobby and invited them into the treatment room, heaviness filled the space.

"Please, make yourself comfortable. So, what's going on with you?" I asked.

"Well," Elsa said, glancing at her husband for support, "we're pretty discouraged. We've been trying to get pregnant since I was twenty-six. Basically, for five years."

"No wonder you're frustrated."

Elsa nodded. "I've had two miscarriages, a year apart, both in the sixth week of pregnancy. The first one was devastating and the second one even more so. I honestly don't know how much more of this I can take."

"Yes, I know firsthand how heartbreaking miscarriages can be."

"Oh, you do?" Elsa asked, her face softening and her eyes tearing up.

"They're way more common than anyone knows. It's such a taboo topic that women going through it feel so alone."

"For a while, I actually thought it might be Rick's fault." She laughed. "I mean, I didn't want to think it was me. But the fertility doctor ran all the tests, and his sperm count, and quality were normal."

I glanced at Rick, whose eyes were irritated slits, and his jaw was clenched as he peered out the window. This was clearly torture for him. I got it—most guys were uncomfortable talking about their sperm, especially in front of another woman who wasn't their wife.

"All my test results were fine—my fallopian tubes were open, and my hormone levels were good. So, on paper, I should have been able to conceive. Still, I was unable to get and stay pregnant." She glanced at Rick, who was expressionless. "So, we decided to take the IVF plunge."

I shared my thoughts about a treatment approach and Elsa was all in. Rick, on the other hand, hadn't said a word the entire time. He just eyed me suspiciously, with his arms crossed tightly over his chest and his leg shaking up and down. His body language broadcasted that he didn't approve of this witch-doctor voodoo stuff. And he was only there because Elsa had dragged him to the appointment.

I wasn't interested in convincing Rick about the efficacy of acupuncture. Instead, I poured my attention into treating Elsa to get her in the best possible shape for IVF. We focused on building her uterine lining and bringing more Qi to her eggs to get them as healthy as possible before retrieval. I tried my best to deflect Rick's annoyed vibes.

The couple was supposed to start the IVF process the month Elsa started seeing me, but while preparing for it, the drugs she was taking to stimulate egg production had triggered the growth of a large ovarian cyst, and they had to wait for it to reabsorb before they could try again.

For Anna, I recommended Chinese herbs to reduce menstrual cramps and stress. After two months of taking herbs to prevent cramping, her cycles were less painful, and her flow a brighter red, a sign that her stagnant blood was moving, and her lining was improving. Because she suffered from low energy, I recommended a thyroid test, which came back at 1.5 mU/L—within normal limits for conception. During her second month of treatment, she had premenstrual twinging in the uterus, sore breasts, and tender nipples—hallmark signs of early pregnancy. Alas, it was not to be that month. It was just PMS, which can frustratingly present like early pregnancy.

Like Anna, Elsa had signs of blood stagnation, including painful periods, painful intercourse while ovulating, and menstrual clots. She also had been diagnosed with endometriosis and ovarian cysts. Her endometriosis had recently been removed by laparoscopy to prepare for her IVF. I put her on the same blood-moving herbs I had recommended for Anna. After taking them for two months, Elsa reported less pain with intercourse around ovulation, which indicated that her cyst was shrinking. All great signs!

After three months of treatment, on December 2, Elsa was elated to share that she finally was pregnant! She complained of cramping, burning, and a hot ache in her uterus, but she wasn't spotting, and her HCG was high and more than doubling. So far, so good. During her first trimester, the RE monitored her with ultrasounds, and she had weekly acupuncture treatments with me to address her anxiety. Who wouldn't be nervous after two miscarriages?

At the end of Anna's third month of treatment, on December 19, she called to tell me that she was pregnant. It happened just two weeks after Elsa got pregnant! The sisters asked me to keep their pregnancies secret from each other. While I'm an expert at keeping confidences—it's my professional duty—it was extra challenging when I treated them both each week. I was thrilled for the sisters and wanted to delight in the news openly. It was so hard to keep quiet about it!

Anna was excited but tormented by nausea. By nine weeks, she was dry-heaving and, at times, vomiting bright yellow-green stomach bile. To quell her nausea, she snacked throughout the day. Her OB/GYN prescribed an anti-nausea medication, which helped but made her feel shaky and anxious. The drug also gave her stomach spasms and flashing lights in her eyes. Who would want to endure ocular disco lights? No surprise that she tried to avoid the medication. By 11 weeks of pregnancy, she backed way off the drug. By 12 weeks, she had only thrown up a few more times. She came in twice a week for acupuncture treatment to manage nausea, as it was the only thing that staved off the queasiness for a few days at a time. She was worn out from being slammed with pregnancy symptoms.

Three and four months into their respective pregnancies, neither sister had shared their news with the other—still! Anna didn't want Elsa to know that it took only three months for her to conceive after Elsa had been trying for almost five years. Elsa didn't want to reveal that she was pregnant only to possibly miscarry again. In fact, she hadn't told anyone in her family about her pregnancy until morning sickness interfered with her dad's birthday celebration.

After munching on some crackers to quell her nausea, she called her dad. "Dad, I'm so sorry I can't make it to your party. But I have good and bad news. Which do you want to hear first?"

"Let's get the bad news over with."

"I have morning sickness."

"Oh, my goodness. That's fantastic news, honey! Guess what?"

"What, Dad?"

"So does your sister."

"What?!"

"It's the best birthday present I could ever imagine." His voice tapered off.

Elsa could tell that her dad was choked up. "I love you, Dad."

After their conversation, Elsa called Anna in tears.

"Hi, Anna. I just wanted to say congratulations!"

"Oh, thanks. I didn't want to tell you because I didn't want to bum you out."

"I'm so happy for you. And I wanted to share some news with you. Your baby will have a playmate and a cousin!"

"What?! You're kidding? I didn't want to tell you about me because I didn't want to make you feel bad. And little did I know…"

They laughed and cried together. It was the best kind of crying.

The fertility doctor wasn't surprised that Elsa was pregnant. During her first appointment with him, he said he couldn't ignore the data indicating increased success with IVF combined with acupuncture. Her husband Rick's reaction, however, was the best. He was instantly converted. He enjoyed telling everyone the story about how he wasn't a believer in acupuncture or Elsa's decision to pursue it, but he was so happy to be proved wrong. Rick's and my working relationship improved immediately. In fact, he apologized for being a skeptical scoundrel during our first appointment. We shared a good belly laugh.

It was good that Elsa came in for anxiety treatments in early pregnancy because at six weeks, the same time that she had previously miscarried, she had so much bleeding that it looked like a full-blown period. She and her husband were petrified. At the fertility doctor's office, they saw on an ultrasound that the baby had a strong heartbeat. Because of her history, and because emotionally she knew she couldn't cope with another miscarriage, Elsa came in twice a week for acupuncture treatments to calm her anxiety. I put her on Chinese herbs known to stop bleeding in early pregnancy.

Even though it's safe to use herbs in early pregnancy if properly prescribed by a trained herbalist, I was still nervous. What if it didn't help and she miscarried anyway? I was on pins and needles, but I didn't let her know.

Pregnancy was also tough going for Anna. I saw her again at 16 weeks, and while her nausea had mostly dissipated, the low-grade queasiness had not. Worse than that, she had an episode of gushing blood, just like her sister. Alarmed, she went to the emergency room. The ER doctor ordered an ultrasound and found that her cervix was closed, the baby had a heartbeat, and the placenta looked great. She had experienced a subchorionic hematoma, where blood accumulates between the fetus or placenta and the uterine lining. As happens sometimes, Anna's body had released the stagnant blood. This is not uncommon in patients with blood stagnation; however, it's terrifying to experience what seems like hemorrhaging. Because the problem resolved quickly, I chose not to put her on herbs.

Elsa continued weekly acupuncture treatments and had frequent ultrasounds. At eight weeks, an ultrasound showed a pool of blood in her uterus the same size as the embryo. Elsa had a subchorionic hematoma, just like her sister. She expelled the dark blood soon thereafter, and the bleeding tapered off. Her baby remained healthy, and the bleeding finally stopped at ten weeks, so I recommended that she stop the herbs.

Elsa had nausea for a few weeks, but she decided to forgo Western drugs. Thankfully, at 12 weeks, her nausea lifted. At the end of her pregnancy, she could eat without difficulty except for a little heartburn. She suffered from cold sores inside her nose, bloody noses, and sinus problems throughout. Pregnancy wasn't the easiest road for the sisters, to say the least.

I didn't see Anna again until she reached 34 weeks. She was still a bit nauseous and had come in for help with swelling and joint pain in her hands and feet. They were so swollen that her knuckles hurt to touch. She was anemic, which is a condition that must be addressed at the end of pregnancy for the health of the mother and the baby. Women lose blood during delivery, so they must have an abundance of red blood cells ahead of time.

Elsa came in on June 28 at 34 weeks. She was worn out and complained of nightmares tormenting her. Once again, her nausea had reared its ugly head, and she was having loose stools. But the most concerning sign was her belly was smaller than it should be for where she was in pregnancy. Her doctor suspected she wasn't retaining enough fluid, and as a result, her amniotic fluid was low. She was put on bed rest for a week with extra fluids. After a week, she measured even smaller than she had the previous week. At 38 weeks, her doctor decided to induce her due to intrauterine growth restriction (IUGR). The safest course was the immediate delivery of her baby. Elsa was admitted that evening and gave birth to her tiny but healthy son the next morning. At birth, Shane was 5 lbs. 1 oz. Luckily, his Apgar score was great, indicating his lungs had developed normally. Lung issues are common in preemies.

When Elsa saw her placenta, it was brown and gray—not colorful like she had read they were supposed to be. She asked the doctor about this, and he said the placenta hadn't initially attached well inside her uterus, resulting in placental insufficiency. The doctor was relieved the baby was safely out of her womb and doing well.

Placental insufficiency means that the organ no longer supplies adequate oxygen and nutrients to the baby from the mother's bloodstream. Without this essential support, the baby cannot grow and thrive. This can lead to low birth weight and premature birth.

On July 24, at 36 weeks, Anna started vomiting again, her hands and knuckles were painful, and her sleep was fitful. She also had cramps that wrapped around her lower back. This time, she welcomed the signs and symptoms because she knew her body was preparing for labor.

Her baby girl was born four weeks after her cousin. I was thrilled for Elsa and Anna and their babies, who would have a beloved cousin, playmate, and friend for life.

WHEN THE TIME IS RIGHT

When Jacey came to see me, she was young—just 26—and healthy. She and her husband enjoyed working out at the gym. In fact, I bumped into them there occasionally. Jacey is hilarious, and we enjoyed bantering before, during, and after her acupuncture treatments. She had shoulder-length dark hair that flowed when she walked, like she starred in a shampoo commercial. Her desk job was good enough, but what she really wanted was a baby.

Jacey had been off birth control pills for a year when she first came to see me. She reported having just one period six months after she had stopped taking them, and she was concerned that something was wrong. Her lack of periods indicated that she was rarely ovulating. When she did ovulate, she would get awful headaches, so I knew her hormones were out of whack.

After one month of acupuncture treatments, she reported having an excruciating headache that spread across her head and centered around her eyes. These are typical of headaches caused by a reaction to estrogen, and I used an effective point combination including points in her elbows and feet to get rid of them. She was disappointed not to be pregnant and to still be getting headaches, but relieved to know she could still ovulate, as evidenced by the headache. This ovulation did not lead to pregnancy, but it did lead to a period, which was a relief after not having them for so long. She felt at least a little bit more normal.

Over the months of treatment, Jacey continued to ovulate and have periods. Her headaches around ovulation slowly vanished as her hormones became more balanced. At this point, her husband told her he did not want to try for a baby anymore. He wasn't interested in changing his lifestyle to fit a baby's needs and liked that they could do whatever they wanted to do whenever they wanted to do it. Despite his sudden realization, Jacey kept trying. Luckily for her, he didn't mind having unprotected sex.

One day, after nine months of treatment, I said to her, "I think you should go see a fertility doctor."

She peered up from the treatment table, frowning. "Why? Do you think I'm a lost cause?"

"Oh, not at all! Western treatments work much better in conjunction with TCM. Trust me, I've seen it work for so many of my patients."

"Really?" The light returned to her eyes. "Oh, thank goodness."

"You've come faithfully for nine months, and we've definitely made progress. We've regulated your periods and alleviated your headaches. While I'm aware these things are beneficial, and I love spending time with you, it's not the primary reason you came to see me."

"Yes, and I'm so thankful. I guess I'll try the fertility doctor."

One of the best parts of my job is chatting with and getting to know my patients, but it's not my social hour. The goal of treatment is to help patients get pregnant and have healthy babies.

Continuing to treat Jacey without results felt a little selfish, especially since she wasn't yet pregnant.

After suggesting she see the RE, I didn't see Jacey for a year and a half. After an emotional regroup as a couple, her husband was back on board with trying to conceive because he knew how important it was to Jacey.

The fertility doctor suggested she come back for acupuncture, since it had regulated her cycles so well in the past. He also suggested she have a laparoscopy to look for endometriosis, which they found and removed. Two months after that surgery, she got a positive pregnancy test, but, sadly, her pregnancy only lasted one week.

Next, Jacey tried a medicated cycle using Clomid, Menopur, and HCG. Clomid is a drug familiar to most women trying to conceive, as it is used to promote ovulation and boost estrogen and progesterone in a cycle. Menopur is an expensive drug used to stimulate the growth of more than one egg at a time. HCG, in addition to being the hormone released during pregnancy, is the trigger shot that ensures ovulation will happen. Jacey had grown ten eggs, but because of her history, they went ahead with an IUI anyway. Fertility clinics usually won't do IUI if a woman produces more than three eggs because of the high risk of multiples. Alas, becoming a reality TV star à la Octomom wasn't in the cards anyway, because it didn't work. They underwent a few more months of fertility treatments but eventually took a break. I was sad for Jacey and wasn't sure if I would see her again.

Three months after her last fertility treatment, and with no acupuncture, Jacey emailed that she had become pregnant naturally!

She was very nauseous during her first trimester and came for acupuncture treatments to help her be able to get food down and keep it down. When stomach Qi goes up, it causes burping, nausea, and vomiting. Acupuncture gently "redirects" it back down, relieving these symptoms. I always know the anti-nausea treatment works when a woman tells me she's hungry by the end of it.

After over three years of trying to conceive, Jacey delivered a gorgeous little girl. After everything they had endured, she and her husband had no interest in trying again. They had hit the jackpot and were ready to be done and just enjoy their darling baby girl.

EGG DONATION: BORROWED EGGS

Sometimes women cannot get pregnant with their own eggs. This is the case for women with very low AMH, premature ovarian failure, or genetic issues that they don't want to pass on to their children.

The beauty of using a donor egg is that the recipient is the biological mother of the baby she's carrying, and if they use his sperm, her male partner is the genetic father. The baby receives all the nourishment that makes up the tissues and blood of its body from its mother who carries it in her womb. The genetics may not be hers, but the biology is.

The genetic blueprint from the donor egg is like the outline of a drawing, but the mother who carries the baby fills in the drawing with her own colors.

For women who want to be pregnant and breastfeed, but can't use their own eggs, this is an elegant solution.

DONOR EGG IVF VIRGIN

In 2004, I had been in practice for five years, and hadn't heard anything about donor egg IVF. In other words, I was a donor egg IVF virgin. So, when Remy came to see me and said she wanted electroacupuncture to prepare her for a donor egg IVF—IVF with her husband's sperm and another woman's egg—I hid my judgment. Being uninformed about donor egg IVF, it seemed like a strange idea. Why would she use someone else's egg? Why can't she use her own egg? Will it still be her baby? I was uninformed and judgmental, though hopefully she didn't notice.

What I learned over the course of her treatment completely changed my mind about donor egg IVF. She told me that, yes, the DNA came from the donor, but the child would be biologically hers. I had never considered this before.

It makes sense, though, that if you put a five-day-old, 200-300 cell blastocyst in its future mother's uterus, it gathers all of its biological material from its mother: all of the blood, cells and tissues it uses to grow into a baby. As baby grows inside her, it hears its mom's voice, feels her heartbeat, and gets all its nutrition from mom. The mother is in control of what goes into her body throughout the pregnancy. When the baby is born, it drinks mother's milk if she's able to breastfeed. Donor egg IVF allows a mother to experience pregnancy who might otherwise not be able to.

Another thing I've learned in practice is that pregnancy doesn't make one a mother. Mothering a child, no matter whose womb it came from, makes one a mother. Some women have a deep desire to carry a child, and for those for whom it is not possible due to age or premature ovarian failure, donor egg IVF is a beautiful solution.

After her baby girl was born, Remy came to see me a few times to help with milk supply issues and the normal stresses that come with new motherhood.

After having her baby, many of Remy's symptoms that were evidence of her high FSH and premature ovarian failure were starting to turn around. Her cycles became more regular, and her hot flashes began to disappear. She was hoping to TTC naturally. This wasn't in the cards for her, however, as her periods slowly started to disappear.

Five years after her first child was born, she was ready for another frozen transfer. We did the pre-IVF transfer protocol again, and again she became pregnant—this time with a boy.

Since then, Remy has come back in as needed, and it's lovely to hear the stories of her growing children. Interestingly, Remy hears that her daughter, Kylie looks a lot like her. This is in part due to the donor she and her husband chose. It's also because her children carry her biology.

Science backs this up. In a study, pony embryos were transferred into thoroughbred mares and thoroughbred embryos were transferred into pony mares. The resulting foals were compared to foals produced from mares of the same breeds, and growth was tracked until all foals reached three years of age. Pony foals carried by thoroughbred mares were larger at birth than pony foals carried by pony mares, and thoroughbred foals carried by thoroughbred mares were larger at birth than thoroughbred foals carried by pony mares.[2]

In 2015, a study pointed to a similar human effect; mothers who use donor eggs may pass some of their genetic material on to their children through their endometrial fluid. This is also true of surrogates who carry another woman's embryo.

Molecules known as MicroRNAs that are secreted in the mother's womb act as a communication system between the mother (or surrogate) and the growing fetus. "The endometrial milk nurtures the embryos, but it is also involved in gene regulation," says Dr. Simon, one of the authors of a study on this topic. "This epigenetic effect begins to happen at the moment of conception," says Dr. Simon. "If you take out the micro-RNA, this regulation disappears."

But it's about more than how your baby will look. Dr. Simon says that this is the beginning of every influence that a mother (or surrogate) can have, including the onset of diseases. For example, if a mother is obese or has Type 2 diabetes at the time of conception, it can directly affect her growing fetus. "The condition of the mother at the time of pregnancy makes a huge difference," says Dr. Simon. "There are many things a mother can change regardless of whether her baby comes from her own eggs or not, and by the same token a surrogate can modify her lifestyle for the baby."[3]

---

2. The influence of maternal size on pre- and postnatal growth in the horse: III Postnatal growth W R Allen, Sandra Wilsher, Clare Tiplady and R M Butterfield
3. https://lehmannhaupt.com/2016/01/06/becoming-a-solo-mom-via-assisted-reproductive-technology-donor-eggs/

Remy's children are now in middle and high school; they are two healthy and happy kids who love robots and forensic science. Remy's son, John, thinks coming from a donor egg is "kind of weird," but otherwise doesn't have any thoughts about it. His mom guesses he doesn't understand how it all works at ten years old, so it's hard to get a real sense of what he thinks. As far as looks and behavior, John looks and acts *just* like his father, Alex, especially from behind and in the way they walk. Their mannerisms are so alike, and they have a very close relationship.

Remy asked Kylie if she feels different coming from a donor egg, and she said no; she doesn't feel any different from anyone else.

Kylie said, "It would be a bigger deal to me if I was adopted, but I'm not, so it's not as big of a deal." Her best friend is adopted, and they have talked about her meeting her birth mother, but Kylie doesn't see similarities. When asked if she is curious about her donor, she said only, "Maybe a little." Her biggest curiosity about the donor is what she looks like and maybe if they share any behavior traits. She has never asked about her donor or the process and seems to only think about it when Remy asks her questions.

Kylie is more curious about her "vanishing twin," as Remy was pregnant with twins until around 12 or 13 weeks. She wondered if it was a boy or a girl. She also asked if she and John were "the same," as in having the same genetic make-up. Remy explained how they were created at the same time, with the same donor, so technically like fraternal twins, just born at different times.

Remy says both kids look like Alex—John more than Kylie. Oddly, they have frequently heard from people how much Kylie looks like Remy and John looks like Alex.

Her cousin once said, "Wow, you each got a mini-me!" (She didn't know about the donor situation.)

Remy wrote in an email:

Sometimes I'll see a photo of Kylie and totally see myself. Maybe that's wishful thinking, though. I guess the one trait that really stands out is that both kids are pretty short (I'm 5'8ish – used to be 5'9" but I'm shrinking...and Alex is barely 5'7"). Kylie has topped out, I think, at 5'1". John is still growing but is quite a bit shorter than friends his age. Our donor was 5'4".

We have always been open about our donor process, and it usually surprises people. I actually like talking about it, as I feel like it normalizes it if we don't make it a big deal and share our story openly.

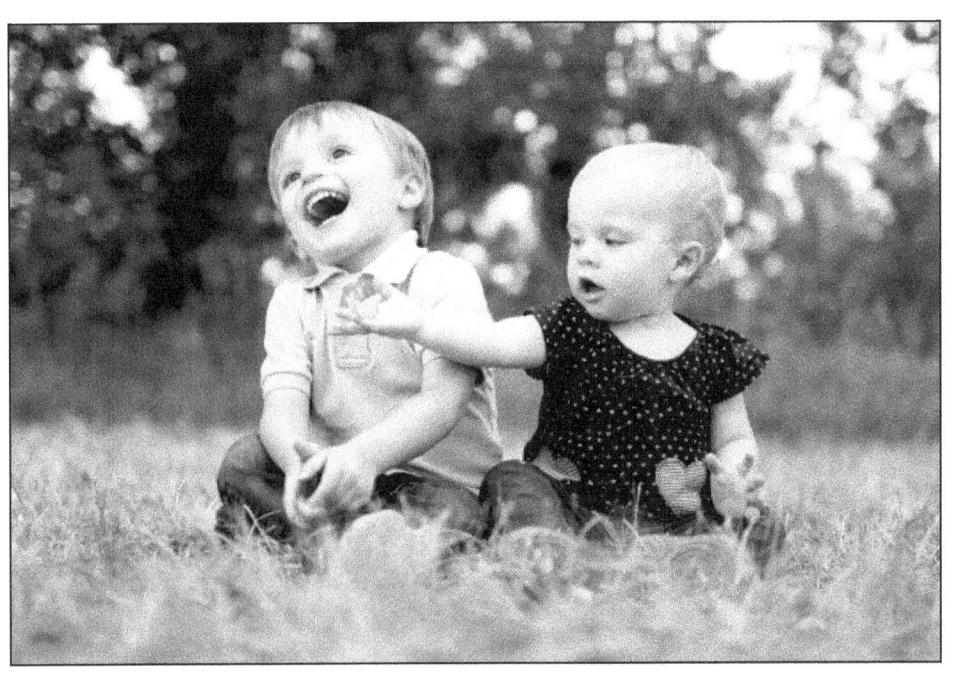

Alana's kids

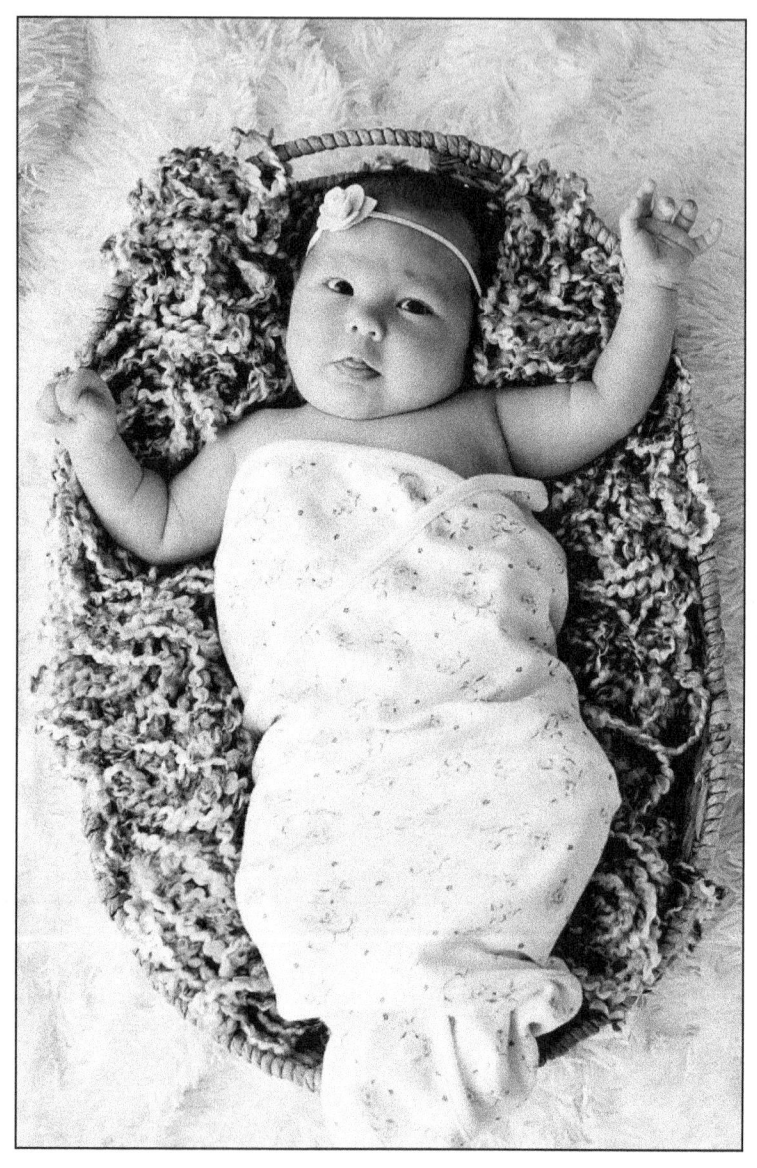

Baby Jade

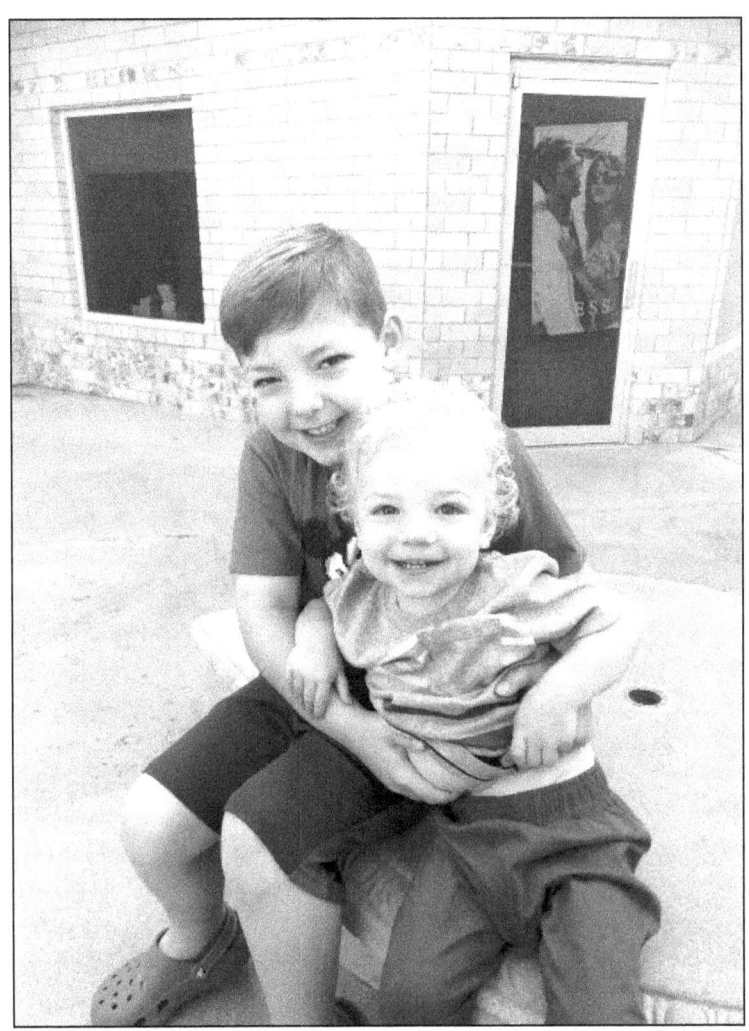

Alisa's boys

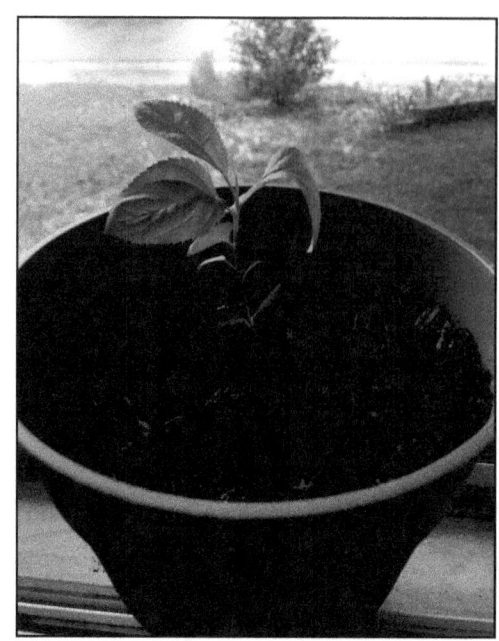

Cora's sapling

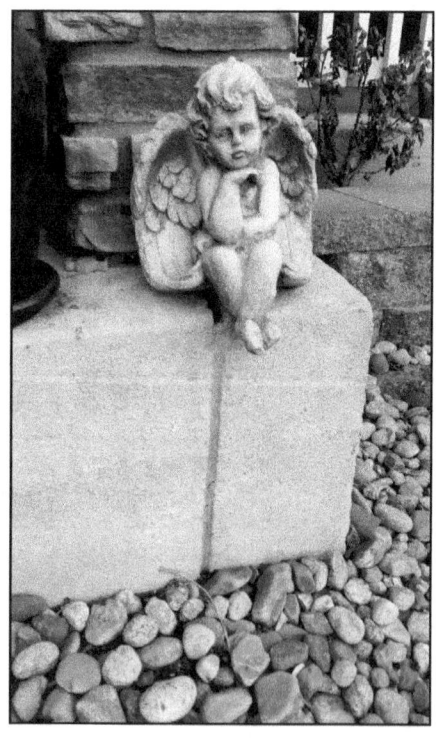

Tyrs statue

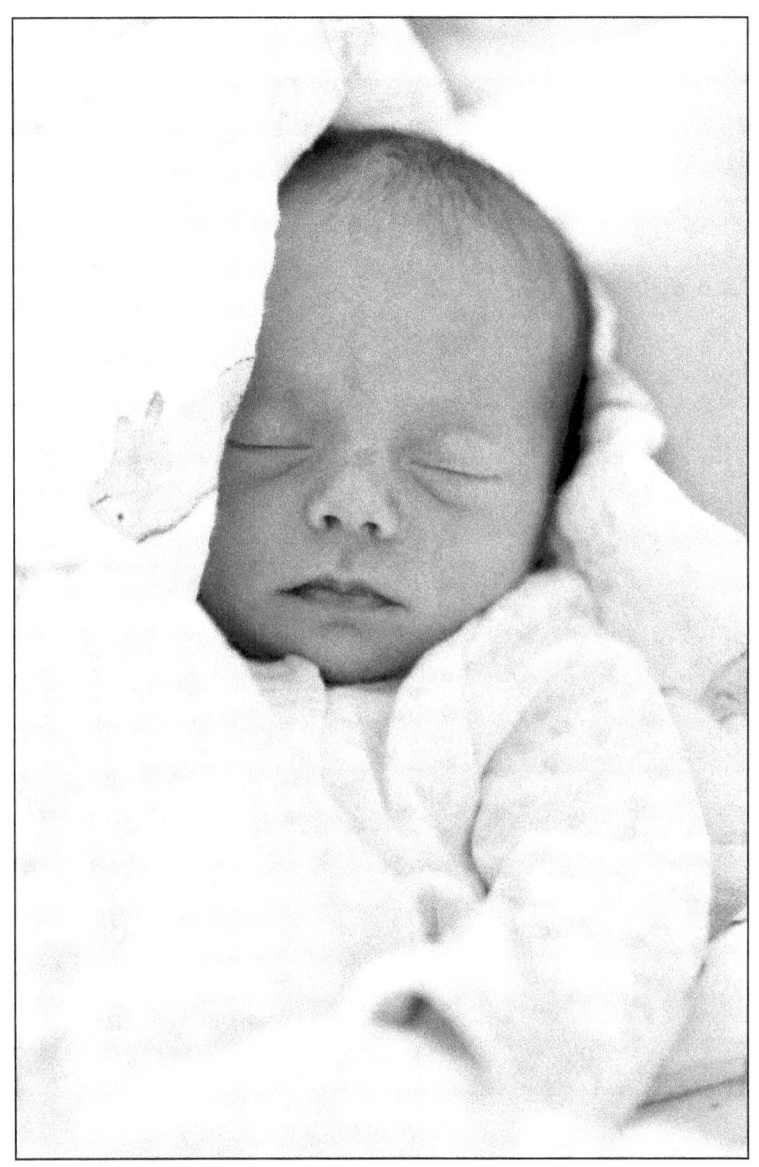

Katrin's baby

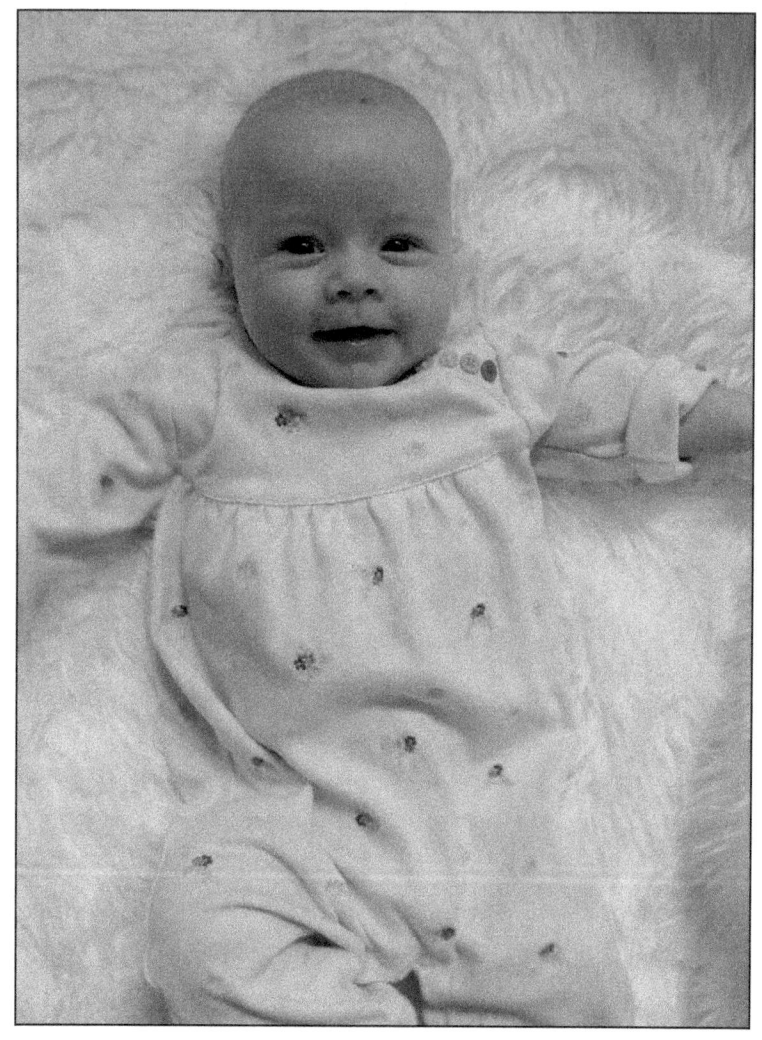

Kylie

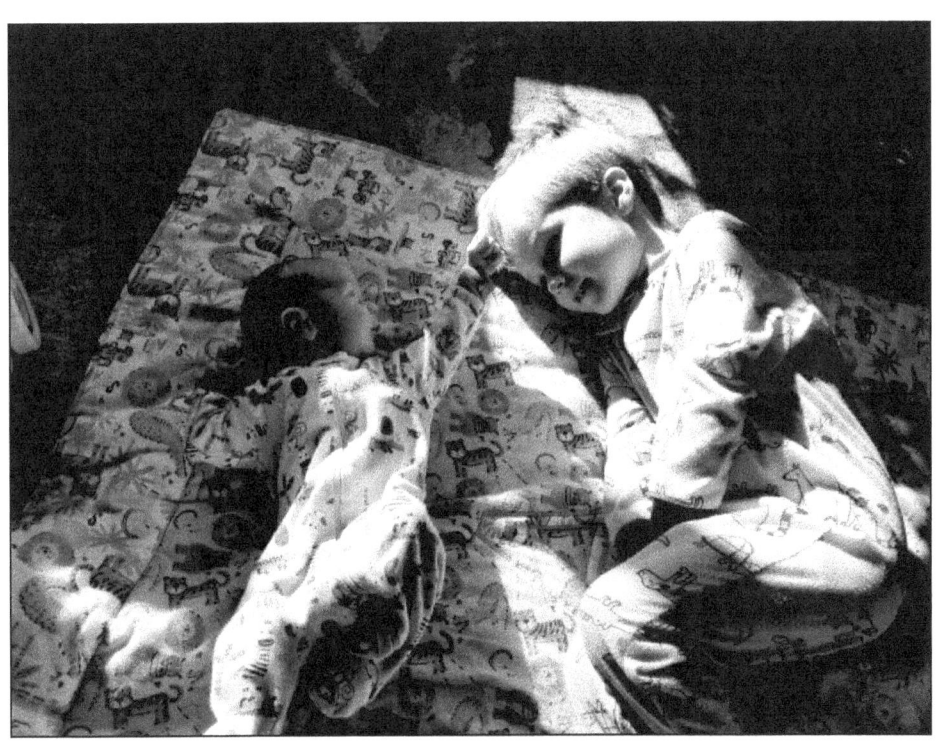

Mary's boys

TRIPLE TREASURE

"It has been three long years of sex on command. My husband has been a good sport, but, honestly, this is killing our sex life," Amanda said, wringing her hands.

"I'm so sorry. Tell me what's going on," I said. Even though I had heard a version of this story many times before, each tale was different; each woman had challenges unique to her.

"Oh, you'll be sorry you asked," she said, laughing. Her laughter was tinged with sadness. "So, here's the lowdown on my reproductive drama. Brace yourself. I have endometriosis and diminished ovarian reserve. I've had a laparoscopy to remove endometriosis, which has helped with my period cramps. I've had two miscarriages in the last two years. I mean, whoever thought it would be this difficult?" She sighed and held my gaze. "I'm not normally a depressed person, but there's only so much a woman can take. And to make matters worse, I'm not sleeping well. I guess you could say I'm a mess."

"That's rough. But you should know you're not alone. Not by any means. If I may ask, when did you miscarry? It will give me important information."

"At nine weeks' gestation and again at five weeks."

"I'm glad you're here." I was anxious to get her up on the table for her first treatment. I knew I could take the edge off and help with her reproductive issues. "Let's first focus on helping you feel better."

Inserting needles in Amanda's arms, legs, and abdomen to move Liver Qi and to calm her Shen, or spirit, helped immensely. After her treatment, Amanda felt lighter emotionally, and her sleep improved.

During subsequent appointments, Amanda told me she was preparing for an IUI with Clomid. This was supposed to be her last time on Clomid, as it gave her visual disturbances, an unsettling side effect. She felt some uterine twinges during the two-week wait of one of her IUI cycles, which meant possible embryo implantation. Unfortunately, an unwelcome visitor arrived on day 28—her period.

Needing a break from the stress of trying to conceive, she stopped acupuncture treatment for a while. When she returned three months later, I prescribed herbs to treat the lingering side effects of Clomid. Her FSH was 15.5—high for a 38-year-old and nearly too high to do IVF with her own eggs. She was quite depressed to hear this.

Amanda had a second laparoscopy to remove more endometriosis, which made her periods less painful. Her optimism returned. Six months after starting acupuncture, her temperature climbed to 99.5 in the middle of her luteal phase, a sign that perhaps an embryo had implanted and was creating HCG, the pregnancy hormone. She even spotted—also a sign of implantation. She wanted to rejoice but took a wait-and-see approach. Cruelly, her period came with a vengeance.

She started weekly acupuncture treatments, and her mood and cramps improved.

Once again, the fertility doctor put her on Clomid, this time with Follistim injections on days three, five, and seven to increase the production of eggs. She became hot again on Clomid but thankfully was spared the visual disturbances. On day 14, she received an HCG trigger shot, as she had one big dominant follicle and four smaller ones. She had an IUI on day 15. During the two-week wait in the mid-luteal phase, she felt uterine twinges again, and her nipples became very sore. Whenever I hear the words "sore nipples" in the luteal phase, especially when it's not a normal symptom for that patient, I feel hopeful that she's pregnant.

Indeed, Amanda was pregnant! Her HCG rose from 127 to 192, which wasn't great, but sometimes HCG starts out slowly. Ideally, HCG levels should double every 48 hours in early pregnancy. The next day it was 325, a slow rise. Trying to remain optimistic, I told Amanda about a patient whose HCG only rose by 75 percent every other day, and she delivered a healthy baby boy.

The day before her 39th birthday, Amanda had an ultrasound that showed a yolk sac, but no heartbeat yet. This is not uncommon, as the heartbeat is usually seen around six weeks. She was only five weeks and six days—one day short of six weeks, but there was room for error. No reason to give up hope yet. Amanda said her pregnancy symptoms were coming and going but weakening.

She miscarried a week later—her third in three years. Amanda was losing hope that she would ever have a baby. Approaching 40 wasn't helping her mental state, either. Fertility in women declines precipitously after age 35.

Her RE advised her to wait two cycles before TTC again, so I put her on herbs to strengthen her after all she had endured. Her hair had started falling out, and she was exhausted. To make matters worse, she had developed jawline acne, a sign that her endometriosis was returning.

Amanda jokingly said, "I'm getting acne like a teen without the benefit of a teenager's fertility."

Amanda had been receiving acupuncture for a year and working with the fertility doctor. Once again, she was prescribed Clomid, which made her sweaty, thirsty, and gave her headaches and insomnia—all signs of internal heat. The cycle didn't work, and she had a third surgery for endometriosis. This time, they found significant endometriosis and cleaned it all out. She waited another month to recover.

She said to me, "What is this? *Groundhog Day*?"

She felt tons better without the rogue endometrial tissue in her abdomen and even felt like having sex again. The next cycle, the RE put her on Clomid and Follistim again, and she produced six follicles! She was triggered with HCG on day 14, and on her ultrasound, they could see that three eggs released. She had an IUI on days 14 and 15. She had sore breasts, but alas, not her nipples this time, and her period came on day 28.

So close, but so far away!

The very next cycle, she repeated the regimen of Clomid and Follistim and released four follicles. All she got for her trouble was ovarian cysts, prompting her to take time off until they reabsorbed. She continued taking herbs to improve her mood, sleep, and blood circulation. She also started a low-inflammation diet, eliminating wheat, red meat, and sugar.

After her cysts resolved, she started Clomid and Follistim again and developed six follicles. Another IUI. Once again, sore nipples! She was tired, nauseous, and light-headed. An ultrasound showed she had lots of corpus lutei on her ovaries, indicating that she had ovulated many eggs.

Amanda returned four months later, announcing, "I'm still unpregnant." She laughed ruefully and said, "It's time for a new approach. It doesn't seem like I will ever be pregnant with my own eggs." She and her husband discussed options with their RE, and they all decided that the best option at this point would be IVF using donor eggs.

Amanda prepared for a donor egg IVF cycle. The donor produced 29 eggs, 16 of which turned into embryos after being fertilized with Amanda's husband's sperm. Ten of the embryos were exceptionally good—a fantastic result. Almost five years after trying to get pregnant, and two years after her first acupuncture treatment, the RE transferred two perfect embryos into her uterus. Then she had to wait. Wait to see if the embryos took. Wait to see if they were viable. Wait to see if she could carry to term.

I didn't see Amanda again for treatment but ran into her several weeks later in the grocery store's produce section. I spotted her rifling through the avocados, looking for the perfect one. I couldn't help but notice her swollen belly.

"Wow! Look at you! Are you about four months?"

She laughed. "Would you believe me if I told you just two and a half months?"

I shook my head. "Everyone's different."

"Especially when they're having triplets!"

"What?!" I covered my mouth.

She held her belly and nodded. "I know! One of the eggs split, so I'm carrying identical twins and their fraternal twin. All boys!"

I shook my head in disbelief. "Oh, my god! But, honestly, three babies at once?!"

"Right now, I'm reveling, but once they're born, I'm sure I'll be reeling from exhaustion." "But it's the good kind of exhaustion—right?"

"Oh, for sure."

Many months later, I emailed Amanda to see how the delivery had gone.

She replied: *My delivery sucked. I had a Cesarean, which was the worst pain of my life. The recovery was unbelievably difficult. I couldn't stand up straight for two months! The kids were born at 30 ½ weeks because one of them had intrauterine growth retardation (IUGR) but he has recovered and is very healthy like the other two. We don't have any learning deficits or anything to be worried about, so I consider us to be extremely lucky.*

About a year later, I invited myself to Amanda's home. I was dying to see the baby boys, and she was gracious enough to let me come visit. The new parents had converted the bottom level of their house into an apartment where the boys could roam without getting into trouble; it was completely baby-proofed. There was a kitchen as well, so bottles and snacks could be made quickly. The entire operation was on a strict routine, so that each baby could get what he needed, and the parents could get a little rest in between. The living room opened out into a big, fenced backyard where the boys could toddle around in a safe, controlled environment—a beautiful solution for their triplets.

THE PERFECT BANANA

Pam was a 32-year-old university professor who dressed like a graduate student just coming in from the library. She came to my office with a messy bun, wearing a clever t-shirt and sweats. She was looking for help after suffering a miscarriage at seven weeks.

When she climbed up on the acupuncture table and reclined, I felt her pulses and they were thin. I asked her to show me her tongue, a key indicator of health in TCM, and saw teeth marks on the sides, as well as a white coating on its surface. Pam complained of fatigue, digestive issues, and excessive worrying. She also had low thyroid values based on a TSH test. These are all classic signs of a weak Spleen in TCM.

The "Spleen" in TCM is a collective group of functions, and not the actual spleen organ. Women with weak TCM Spleens often suffer from recurrent miscarriage, as well as hormonal imbalances (especially PMS), heavy periods, and easy bruising.

Professors and others who rely heavily on their brains for work must find ways to balance their lives so that overthinking doesn't damage their TCM Spleens. Students who throw themselves into studying all the time without balancing it out with Spleen-friendly behaviors are symbolically eating cake with both hands. It's too much at once.

Spleen-friendly behaviors include daily exercise, but not to the point of exhaustion; small meals at regular times; no iced or cold foods or drinks; no raw foods; and mindfulness meditation to quiet the monkey mind.

When food and drink are warm and cooked, it allows the energy that one would use to digest challenging things, like a bowl of salad and a large, iced drink, to instead go to the reproductive system, where it is needed for fertility.

Pam stopped trying to conceive for a couple of months and continued weekly acupuncture treatments for four months to get her body healthy and back in balance. She reported having more regular menstrual cycles. Where previously, some months she would ovulate erratically on day 10 or day 17, after three months of treatment, she began ovulating on day 13 or 14, which is much better for conception.

Why does the day of ovulation matter? To help my patients understand the process, I tell them to imagine that eggs are like bananas. A day 10 egg is like a green banana—less mature—and the uterine lining is often less ready to accept an embryo even if the egg is fertilized. An egg released on day 14 is like a perfect, yellow banana. An egg released on day 17 or after is like a spotty, overripe banana. Even if it can be fertilized, the egg's DNA is beginning to break down, and the uterine lining might not receive the embryo because other hormone-dependent processes could be past their prime.

You may know someone (it could even be you) who has become pregnant with an egg ovulated earlier or later than the optimal time. In my own case, based on early ultrasounds to confirm and date my pregnancy, it seems my daughter was a day nine egg. It is possible.

Acupuncture regulates the hypothalamic-pituitary-ovarian (HPO) axis, making it possible for the egg to be released at the best time for fertilization, somewhere between days 13-15. When you are being repeatedly stuck with tiny needles, such as during acupuncture, endorphins are released into your system to help you deal with the pain. But since acupuncture really isn't painful when done by an acupuncturist with the proper training, you just get to enjoy your endorphins. Most patients describe feeling blissful during their treatments because of the release of endorphins. These endorphins communicate with the hypothalamus, pituitary and ovaries, regulating your menstrual cycle, and even improving your chances of conception.[4]

I treated Pam with points over her uterus and ovaries, as well as some in her wrists, ankles, and feet to balance her hormones. I gave her all the Spleen dietary advice, which, as a good student, she followed completely. She also took a thyroid medication to balance her thyroid levels. After four months of weekly acupuncture treatments and taking herbs that bolstered Pam's Spleen, she became pregnant! She stopped treatments during her pregnancy, but I later learned she had a healthy baby girl in March of 2015.

Two years later, Pam came to see me again after trying to conceive for six months with no luck. Her thyroid had developed antibodies to itself, and she now had Hashimoto's thyroiditis. This condition

---

4 (J Endocrinol Invest. 1989 Nov;12(10):693-8. doi: 10.1007/BF03350035. Oocyte fertilization in vitro is associated with high follicular immunoreactive beta-endorphin levels F Facchinetti 1, P G Artini, M Monaco, A Volpe, A R Genazzani)

adds another layer of difficulty in getting pregnant. Hashimoto's is treatable with supplemental thyroid hormone and a gluten-free, low-inflammation diet. Pam had seen a couple of different functional medicine doctors and was following a strict autoimmune diet that they had prescribed for her, as well as the thyroid medication she had been on before. These seemed to help immensely, and she admitted she felt much better. However, she was now 35, and feeling the pressure to get pregnant again before it was too late.

Two months after restarting acupuncture, she went to a fertility doctor and had an intrauterine insemination (IUI), but it didn't work. She immediately started another medicated IUI cycle, but her lining was only 6.95mm thick, which is a bit low for success (8mm is the bare minimum). As expected, it didn't work. She had an in vitro fertilization (IVF) consultation with a different doctor in Colorado Springs, then another consultation with a different clinic that was twice as expensive. During this time, Pam remained proactive with her self-care and started abdominal massage.

Six months into her treatment with me, she decided to go ahead with the fertility doctor in Colorado Springs. The doctor tested her husband Jim's semen, and found two suboptimal values. The doctor also ran a chromatin test that showed poor sperm quality. One explanation for this could have been that Jim was training for an Ironman race. As someone who was once fairly addicted to running, I understood the drive for strenuous exercise. However, the internal heat levels that result during rigorous training, not to mention the hours sitting on a bike seat, can damage sperm. I suggested that Jim stop training, suspecting it would fall on deaf ears. Achieving that level of fitness is hard-won, and not many would opt to dial it back.

Meanwhile, Jim and Pam went forward with IVF. Her uterine blood flow looked good, and she had a decent number of follicles for a 36-year-old. The number of follicles is important because only about 50 percent of follicles fertilize, and then only about 50 percent of the fertilized ones make it. If you start with eight eggs, you may only end up with two embryos. Hopefully, they are both healthy. The more follicles you have, the better your chances of a live birth.

Unfortunately, Pam became very sick with a respiratory virus during the IVF cycle, and even with all of the exogenous hormones and stimulation medicines she was taking, her hormones dropped, and her follicles weren't growing. She had such a poor response, they had to put the IVF on hold. The fertility doctor insisted that the illness didn't affect her egg quality, but, from a TCM standpoint, it certainly didn't help.

The following month she was feeling much better and started the IVF process again. Everything was looking good. Pam had another relapse of her virus, but the IVF cycle moved forward. The first cycle produced only one follicle, so it was cancelled. In the second cycle, she received the maximum dose of meds, and she produced 11 follicles. Only three were mature, and the one embryo created didn't make it. Her final IVF with her own eggs produced two day 5 blastocysts, but they were both genetically abnormal, so neither were transferred.

Was it possible Pam's eggs weren't viable?

She and the RE began discussing using donor eggs. Pam was on board but wanted to use a donor from Spain instead of the U.S. She had done lots of research and learned that Spain had the best combination of high success rates, low prices, and as a bonus, it was a place that they wanted to visit. Donor egg IVF in the U.S. isn't cheap, at around $30,000 per cycle, so this was a great solution. In Spain it would be closer to $10,000 plus flights.

Pam and Jim traveled to Spain in July of 2018 to start the donor egg process. Their donor produced plenty of eggs, and they created many embryos. They tried two different IVF transfers, one in July of 2018 and one in October of 2018, both of which failed. This was unexpected and very disappointing. Donor egg embryos are usually quite robust, as the donor is young, and her eggs are healthy.

They chose a new donor in February of 2019, and this time they transferred two embryos—no more messing around! Pam got pregnant this time, but only for a few days. Her human chorionic gonadotropin (HCG) never rose much, and ultimately, she miscarried. If you are keeping count, Pam had three egg retrievals in the U.S. with her own eggs, with no embryos available to transfer. Then three donor egg retrievals in Spain which resulted in three transfers, all of which failed.

What was going on?

Needless to say, 2018 was miserable for Pam. Not only was her dream to expand her family going nowhere fast, but also, she and her husband and daughter passed around viruses all year, and her back kept going out. She was ready for a reboot!

The best part about using a Spanish donor was that Pam traveled to the coast of Spain many times that year and was required to stay on bed rest for several days after her transfer. As she waited for each transfer to take, she spent her days gazing out of her window at the azure-colored Mediterranean Sea. She ate fresh Spanish food like seafood paella every day. This was healing to her soul. She said she felt like she had come home.

After returning to Colorado, Pam saw me again in August of 2019 and revealed that she had become pregnant naturally! We were both so excited, thinking this could finally be her reward for so much suffering. Devastatingly, she miscarried just before nine weeks, which was a cruel blow. I can only imagine the pain she went through, because I, too, was a mess when she shared the news.

She and Jim went to a new RE who ordered more fertility testing. Pam and Jim were starting to feel like they were involved in a never-ending science project! This time Jim was the focus. The RE explained that Jim had a balanced translocation that negatively affected his sperm quality. In a balanced translocation, a piece of a chromosome is broken off and attached to another one in such a way that it did not affect Jim's growth and development as a child. However, when his sperm cells divide, they can end up with extra genetic material or missing genetic material, or they can divide normally, which is how they had their daughter. When a sperm with the incorrect amount of genetic material manages to fertilize an egg, it leads to miscarriage, depending on which chromosome and genes are affected. It seemed it wasn't the Ironman training after all—a good thing because it was his passion. Pam was now 38 years old, not necessarily too old to conceive, but she had low fertility markers. She was running out of time and hope. But she didn't give up.

Feeling defeated, but like they wanted to keep going, they went forward with yet another IVF and a local donor. Unlike with the

Spanish donors, Pam and Jim had access to her information, including photos, hobbies, and lifestyle, and they loved her. If Pam couldn't provide the eggs herself, this local donor was the next best thing. In Spain, the couple was in the dark about the donor, because in Spanish IVF clinics, the clinic staff matches the patient with the mother's likeness. The American donor produced an abundance of eggs, 22 of which were frozen.

In October of 2019, just before the donor's egg retrieval, Pam learned that she was again pregnant naturally! She and Jim decided to retrieve and freeze the donor's eggs just in case, especially with her history of miscarriage. Pam had a private and tranquil pregnancy during the global pandemic. In June of 2020, she delivered a beautiful little girl who looks just like her big sister. Pam is grateful the Spanish IVFs did not work out; otherwise, she might not have her baby girl.

The 22 frozen donor eggs have since been released to another hopeful mother-to-be. The price tag for Pam and Jim's fertility work came to around a whopping $120,000! The irony is her second baby girl was free.

EMBRYO ADOPTION: SNOWFLAKE ADOPTION

"Snowflake" or embryo adoption is the term used when a woman or a couple adopts the frozen embryo of another couple who has gone through IVF. It is a beautiful solution for women who would like to be pregnant but aren't concerned that the genetics of the baby aren't hers or her husband's. Like with donor eggs, the baby takes its nourishment and biology from the mother carrying it, even though they don't share genetics. The mother carrying the child controls what she puts into her body, making it a healthy vessel for the embryo. She can experience pregnancy and breastfeed her baby if she chooses.

This is also a wonderful option for couples who have created more embryos using IVF than they plan to use themselves. They can select the family who will receive their embryos and feel at peace knowing their genetic offspring will be part of a family who cherishes them.

SNOWFLAKE BABY

When Alana came to see me, her dream to become a mother was vanishing. All her friends, also in their early thirties, were getting pregnant easily, whereas she had been diagnosed with diminished ovarian reserve. Three dreaded words for a woman who wants children. Most women's fertile years wane at around 45, so to be told you are done at 31 is devastating. This condition affects nearly one-third of infertility patients and refers to a decrease in the quality and quantity of eggs in a woman's ovaries. In other words, Alana's eggs had reached their expiration date.

At around 5'8", Alana was fit and healthy with shoulder-length light brown hair. Women with diminished ovarian reserve don't look unhealthy or any different from fertile women. It's a mystery why this happens. Chinese medicine considers *jing*—the reserves that a woman gets from her parents—to be the culprit with low ovarian reserve. Poor *jing* reserves lead to premature ovarian failure and diminished ovarian reserve. Women and men can burn through their *jing* with sex, drugs, and rock 'n' roll. In other words, living in excess. They can also deplete it by burning the candle at both ends. I suspect the second was Alana's case, as she was a driven and successful medical professional and had, no doubt, burned the midnight oil for years. However, there was likely some other underlying issue, as I have treated plenty of high-performing doctors who have children with their own eggs.

Alana and her husband, Steven, had been trying to conceive for three and a half years. She had endometriosis with spotting for two to eight days before each period, painful ovulation, and painful periods. She had tried two rounds of medicated IUI, and one round of IVF, all of which failed. Her job as a veterinarian was stressful, causing her to have gastric ulcers. Her AMH tested low at 0.69 ng/mL (normal for her age is 2.1 ng/mL), not hopeless, but low for her age.

IVF using a donor egg from a younger woman was still an option, but Alana had decided against this, and had moved straight to "snowflake" or embryo adoption. The embryos of these procedures are referred to as "snowflake babies" because they're still frozen on dry ice when they are adopted. When couples use IVF to get pregnant, they often have embryos remaining after they finish having children. Embryo adoption allows the family with remaining embryos to select a family for them. The adopting family uses the donated embryos to achieve pregnancy and give birth to their child. The beauty of a snowflake adoption is that a woman who is told she can't get pregnant is able to carry, deliver, and breastfeed her baby. Whereas a child adopted after birth might have been exposed to chemicals, alcohol, and drugs in utero, a woman carrying a donated embryo can choose what she puts in her body.

In Alana's case, the original parents of her adopted embryos were older and had had their own fertility issues. The eggs came from an anonymous young donor, while the sperm came from the husband. In 1997, they created 12 embryos and transferred five (!)

into the mother, and the original parents had boy/girl twins. Five is a remarkable number, as these days, a fertility doctor won't transfer more than two. They felt their family was complete, so they decided to put the other seven embryos up for snowflake adoption.

When Alana and her husband adopted the seven remaining embryos, the twins from that same group of embryos were 19 years old and living in Los Angeles. That meant their frozen fraternal siblings had been on ice for 20 years! Everyone prayed that the defrosting would be successful. Freezing techniques have changed a lot over the past 20 years, and not all thaws are successful. The doctor that created and froze the embryos back in 1997 still worked at the same fertility clinic in California, and he recommended that they thaw all the embryos prior to considering a transfer to see if they were still viable. He had never worked with embryos that old, so he was skeptical they would have even one viable embryo to transfer.

In November 2016, they thawed all seven embryos. Five didn't make it, but the other two were refrozen as day 5 blastocysts. They were cryopreserved rather than slow-frozen like they had been in 1997, so the chance of survival at the next thawing and transfer into Alana's uterus would be greatly improved. Alana and her husband transferred one of the two embryos a few weeks later.

It worked! Alana became pregnant with a son they named Tyler.

From Alana's blog, August 2017:
I am forever infertile. Having a baby via embryo adoption does not change this. For those of you in that camp with me, I get you. You get me. I love my son dearly and consider him my own, but I

cannot change who God has made me. I am infertile. And for once, I don't need to change this fact. I spent the last four years trying to change this, fighting the reality with so many tests, procedures, and prayers. But now, God is bringing me the peace I have prayed for so many times. Tyler is mine; he is of my flesh and blood—I grew him from a few cells to the baby he is now in my own body, sharing oxygen and blood and life with him. God has entrusted him to our care, and regardless of how he got here, he is our son. As I settle into motherhood, I cannot help but look back on the rocky road that brought me here. For this child I prayed, and God has granted me the gift of motherhood. He did not change my identity in Him, or the fact that I am infertile, but He made a beautiful story out of it all.

When her son was a year old, Alana returned to my office. I was thrilled to see her on the schedule; I enjoyed treating her and was excited to help her prepare for what I assumed was another frozen embryo transfer.

"It's so good to see you! Oh, my goodness! Your baby is so cute! He's such an amazing miracle!"

We looked at photos of baby Tyler on her phone.

"Speaking of miracles…I'm pregnant!"

"What? Naturally?"

She nodded excitedly.

"How?" *Her eggs weren't supposed to be working! And how did she have time for sex with a baby and a job?*

We laughed and probably cried a little, too.

"Maybe my pregnancy primed the pump!"

"Wow! I've never heard of a case of pregnancy curing premature ovarian failure."

We discussed that she must have been meant to have three children, not just two! Even though she now had Tyler and was pregnant with her second baby, she planned to transfer the remaining embryo later, as she and her husband had adopted it, and didn't want to abandon it.

At the time of this writing, she was 13 weeks pregnant with a healthy baby girl. Here is the latest excerpt from Alana's blog:

I'm pregnant! I never thought I would say this without going through months of planning, saving up, ordering medications, injections, flights to California, and doctors' visits. I never thought I would see a second line on the pregnancy test without all the effort that I have come to associate with even having a chance at conceiving. Yet here I am, 12 weeks pregnant! God truly went above and beyond my wildest dreams!

So, here's the story…I went to my annual well-woman exam on October 8th. My doctor gave me a lecture about how, even though we had been trying for over five years to have a baby and only achieved a pregnancy via embryo adoption, it was still possible that I could conceive. She recommended birth control.

I said, "Not to be non-compliant, but I will take my chances…I know they are low, but I would rather not go on birth control."

Well, fast forward 28 days, and my period was a day late. As Tyler and I took an evening stroll around the neighborhood after dinner, I remember praying to God that, no matter the outcome, I would give Him all the glory. And, perhaps for the first time ever, I truly meant it in this context. I would give Him the glory, whether I had many more years of unsuccessful cycles, or if He chose to grant us another child.

It is extremely rare that my period is late, so the next morning I took a cheapo pregnancy test (expired, by the way—from before Tyler). I placed the test on the shelf in the bathroom and sat in the quiet of the early morning reading my morning devotional. When I turned around to look at the test, I truly never expected to see a second line, and yet there it was, plain as day! Not a "squinter," no denying it! I was speechless. I walked out of the bathroom and silently handed the test to Steven.

"Your eggo is preggo?!" he said, giving me a big hug. "Wow! Your heart is pounding."

"Well, of course!"

We were astonished that pregnancy had restored her body to a fertile state. Her daughter, Hannah, was born in 2019, healthy and perfect—a true miracle. And like a snowflake, one in a million.

EGG DONATION: THE GIVING EGGS

Egg donation is a generous act in which a young woman with vibrant, healthy eggs donates them to a woman unable to use her own eggs for pregnancy. Women choose to do this for reasons ranging from financial compensation, wanting to help a friend or family member, or because they simply have a generous nature.

Women turn to egg donation when they can't get pregnant with their own eggs. They may have reached menopause or have poor egg or embryo quality with previous IVF attempts. The most common reason women choose egg donation is poor egg quality due to advanced maternal age. A woman's egg quality declines significantly after age 37.

When a young woman decides to become an egg donor, it's not as easy as just handing over her eggs. The donor must inject herself with drugs and hormones to grow many more eggs than she would normally ovulate in a cycle. The fertility doctor then extracts the eggs from her body—also not a comfortable experience.

The young woman receives financial compensation and the fulfilling feeling that she helped build a family where it otherwise might have been impossible.

IS SOMETHING WRONG WITH MY EGGS?

When Jenny came to see me for treatment, she was 26 years old and struggling to get pregnant. She had quit taking birth control pills five months earlier, but no luck. She wondered what was wrong and worried about her eggs.

She had donated eggs when she was 22, so she could help women with their dream of starting a family. This selfless act was in keeping with Jenny's generous personality. She was always looking for ways to help others. The first time she donated, the doctor retrieved 17 eggs. She couldn't recall the exact number the second time she donated eggs, but she said it was a lot.

But Jenny was wondering if her altruism had backfired. She was concerned that donating eggs might have affected her ability to get pregnant. She was also nervous because the recipients of her eggs were unable to get pregnant, despite having so many of them. She wondered, *is something wrong with my eggs?*

A super fit and healthy young woman, Jenny exercised up to six days a week, including running, yoga, weights, and golf. Her diet was clean; she avoided foods that caused inflammation like wheat, dairy and refined sugar, and she ate plenty of fruits and vegetables.

Her AMH was 2.6 ng/ml, a perfect measure of egg reserve. The normal range of AMH is between 1-3 ng/ml. OB/GYN and fertility doctors measure AMH to assess a woman's ovarian reserve or egg count. According to that number, Jenny still had plenty of eggs left. But were they viable? Our treatment focus was on ensuring they were of good quality.

After determining that she wasn't allergic to bees, I advised her to take royal jelly, a honeybee secretion that is fed to larvae and queen bees for their growth and development. It has antioxidant and anti-inflammatory properties which improve the health of the reproductive system, especially eggs (and even sperm). The natural plant estrogens in royal jelly give a gentle boost to fertility. Worker bees feed royal jelly to the developing queen honeybee larva so when she is fully grown, she can lay up to 2,000 eggs a day. Not that we wanted Jenny to produce that many eggs!

We also did weekly acupuncture treatments to increase her fertility. When treating fertility, my focus is on bringing more blood and Qi (the body's natural energy) to the reproductive system. I also move blood and Qi, especially if they are stuck in these areas. Stuck Qi and blood in terms of fertility issues can cause menstrual cramps and other pain in the lower abdomen. I treat these issues by inserting tiny needles over the ovaries and uterus, and often over the sacral area. I also include points in the wrists, lower legs, and feet, all of which are critical for fertility.

After just one month, Jenny was pregnant. She continued to see me during her pregnancy for nausea and hip pain. I treated her right before delivery to help relax her cervix and prepare emotionally for her first labor and delivery. Acupuncture releases endorphins into the body which makes the patient feel peaceful and calm. I'd like to think that talking with my patients also helps soothe them before their big day.

At long last, her dream came true, and she gave birth to a healthy baby boy!

Jenny came to see me 19 months later when she was overdue with her daughter. We did a relaxing, cervix-opening treatment, and within a few days, she delivered a healthy baby girl.

A little over three years later, she returned, which delighted me, because I loved treating her. She had always responded beautifully to acupuncture—it took almost no time for her to get results from my treatments. She was ready to conceive her third child, and repeating the treatment we had done before, it took just three weeks.

Unfortunately, she miscarried at 8½ weeks. We were both surprised and heartbroken. She passed it on her own with no need for a D&C, the procedure that clears out tissues remaining in the uterus after a miscarriage to prevent infection or heavy bleeding.

Jenny needed a break from trying to conceive, so she took two months off. She returned for treatment during the third month. Not surprisingly, she was quickly pregnant again. Jenny was a bit more nervous this time, so she opted to see me almost weekly through the first trimester to support the pregnancy and calm her anxiety. It was rougher than the previous pregnancies with more nausea and vomiting. Acupuncture helped take the edge off.

In December, a little before Christmas, Jenny delivered a healthy baby boy. She now feels that her family is complete.

THE GREAT GIVEAWAY

At our first appointment, Julie greeted me with a beaming smile that quickly vanished as she shared her story. At 27, she figured she wouldn't have any problem getting pregnant. She had been off birth control for six months, and she and her husband had been trying to conceive with no luck.

"I only took the pill for two months. Before that, my cycles were normal—twenty-nine days, but now they're more like thirty-three to forty days." Then she looked out the window and sighed. "I'm worried that something I did may have affected my ability to get pregnant."

"Oh? What was that?" I asked, my notepad balanced on my lap and my pen in position to jot down this critical information.

"Well, eight months ago, I donated fifty eggs. The woman who received my eggs had a healthy pregnancy. Do you think the egg donation compromised my ability to get pregnant?" She shook her head. "Wouldn't that be ironic if I needed someone else's eggs to get pregnant myself?"

I hoped for her sake this wasn't the case. "I doubt egg donation would compromise your ability to conceive. May I see the report from the RE?"

"Oh, sure." She handed me the readout detailing her fertility stats.

"Okay, great news. Your AMH level is high normal, which indicates a large reserve of eggs."

"Thank goodness!"

"But…"

"Oh, no, here it comes," said Julie, worried again.

"Based on the symptoms you reported—uncomfortable fluid in your abdomen for a few weeks afterward—you suffered from ovarian hyper-stimulation syndrome, or OHSS. Donating fifty eggs at one time is hard on the body, and OHSS is an exaggerated response to the excess hormones you took. OHSS causes the ovaries to swell and become painful. So, even though you still have plenty of eggs left, your body is tired, and you need to heal before you can conceive."

She laughed. "So weird that I helped someone with their fertility and now I need help myself."

After Julie's first month of acupuncture, her cycle shortened to 31 days, a sign that things were heading in the right direction. Her second and third cycles after starting acupuncture were 29 days, the perfect cycle length for fertility, but still no pregnancy. The fourth cycle stretched out to 32 days. This was a disappointing setback.

I suggested Julie go gluten-free to address her chronic digestive issues. Gluten can cause inflammation, which sometimes interferes with fertility in both women and men. Things went downhill from there, and her fifth cycle after starting acupuncture was 42 days. She reported being very tired. What was going on? Was it her gluten-free diet? Work stress? Something else?

Julie's friend, Jenny, who had referred her to me, had also donated eggs around the same time, and she was pregnant after only one month of acupuncture!

Despite her frustration, Julie persevered and ovulated on day 14 during her sixth and seventh cycles. Her periods started on the 28th day—exciting that she was regular, but she had had enough periods. She wanted to be pregnant. She made an appointment with the fertility doctor, as she was ready for the big guns.

During her eighth cycle, after having started acupuncture and herbs, and doing an IUI with medication, she ovulated on day 15. A week later, she began having what she described as weird heart pain. Though this isn't a typical sign of early pregnancy, it was for Julie!

Her pregnancy was successful, and she delivered a healthy baby girl at a little over 40 weeks. Two years later, Julie had a son without Eastern or Western medical interventions. She was delighted and relieved that donating eggs hadn't compromised her ability to have her own children.

ADOPTION: BABIES FROM THE HEART

In my opinion, the most selfless act of a woman is to give up the baby she gestated for nine months and then delivered. Adopting the baby is the second most selfless act. Why? Because of the attachment one feels while carrying that child, as well as the grief at having to give it up—it's not an easy decision.

Although the lucky family who receives the baby desperately wants to raise it and give it a loving home, adoptive parents face unique questions and challenges. They may wonder, *can we love someone else's child, and will the child love us in return*? They must take a leap of faith while facing anxiety about the unknown. While biological children share their parents' genetic make-up and are therefore usually familiar, adoptive children may feel like a mystery with a different set of looks, traits, and characteristics that emerge over time.

Challenges include other people's curiosity about a child that may not resemble the parents, especially if the child has a different ethnicity or race. Questions about an adopted child's background can seem meddling and insensitive, but the best way for adoptive parents to handle this is with patience and grace. They can turn such incidents into teachable moments.

MORE BEAUTIFUL THAN WE CAN IMAGINE

Natasha was 30 years old, a college professor and an avid rock climber. She and her husband, Anthony, often climbed with my husband, Scott, so I knew her from dinners and get-togethers. Natasha and her husband tried to conceive for a year after she went off birth control pills. At the one-year mark, they decided to consult with a gynecologist. She didn't feel desperate or any pressure to have her own biological child but thought she should get checked out anyway.

While Natasha checked out okay, the fertility doctor discovered that Anthony's testicle had a varicocele—a vein enlargement, like a varicose vein. Trauma to the scrotum, typically from a sports injury, is often a culprit. Anthony had been a baseball player and had been hit a few times without a protective cup. Ouch! Varicoceles are a common cause of low sperm quality, which can lead to problems conceiving.

While Anthony had surgery to remove the varicocele, Natasha wasn't interested in going to great lengths to make a baby happen. She had seen a friend pour scads of money and energy into fertility treatments, only to give birth to a baby at 22 weeks. The baby didn't make it because it was too premature, which devastated her friend. As a result, Natasha decided that extensive and expensive fertility treatments, like IVF, weren't for her.

Natasha's openness to adoption was rooted in a childhood experience. When Natasha was eight years old, she had a Siamese cat named Whiskers whom she claimed was the meanest cat ever. No one wanted to visit or house-sit for her family because, like a wild cougar on the loose, the cat would attack any stranger who entered their home. They bred Whiskers with a male Siamese cat, and she gave birth to a purebred litter that was stillborn.

Down the street, there was an orphaned newborn orange tabby kitten whose mother was hit by a car. The owners of the orange tabby gave the kitten to Whiskers, and her whole personality changed. She adored the kitten, cleaning him from head to toe every day. She even started being nice to strangers! From this experience, Natasha learned that mothering wasn't about being pregnant, and being pregnant didn't make you a mother.

Natasha and Anthony started the process of adopting a baby. She felt very strongly that this was the right thing for them. A year and a half later, they were matched, and in November of 2003, they went to Korea to bring their daughter home. When they first met five-and-a-half-month-old Charlotte, they had an instant connection with her, and knew they had made the right decision.

By the time Charlotte was a year old, despite having been off birth control pills for over four years, Natasha still wasn't pregnant. They hadn't been actively trying, but they weren't preventing pregnancy either, as they wanted another child. She and Anthony again started the process of adopting, but this time it didn't feel right. Natasha worried that she couldn't possibly love another child as much as she loved Charlotte. Nevertheless, they went forward with it.

As they were going through the adoption process, Natasha had an incredibly vivid dream of her family posing under a tree for photos with everyone dressed in white button-down tops and jeans. Under the tree, Natasha had Charlotte in her lap, and standing over her shoulder was a blond, blue-eyed boy. *Huh?* Natasha woke up confused. They hadn't even considered a domestic adoption, so how could they have a Caucasian boy? Natasha was at peace with not giving birth; however, her dream was so real it was hard to shake. She chalked it up to wishful dreaming.

Around this time, Natasha had heard that I specialized in fertility acupuncture. Even though we were already friends, she hadn't known about my specialty. She decided to give acupuncture a try.

In the nine months that I treated Natasha, I would insert needles either over her ovaries and uterus, or her sacrum, as well as in her wrists and ankles. Needle placement varied depending on the week, and where she was in her menstrual cycle. I also recommended herbs to improve egg quality and reduce menstrual cramps. Then we would sit together and chat about life.

She got pregnant twice during our work together; however, she miscarried both times, and one of those pregnancies was twins. She stuck it out with me for nine months because she realized she could actually get pregnant. She was amazed, because before starting treatment, she had never been able to get pregnant. But, at the end of that nine-month period, she felt done with treatment. I agreed and said she had given it a very fair chance.

Little did we know that she was pregnant at the time she quit treatment.

Natasha passed the six-week, the eight-week, and the ten-week mark and was still pregnant. Natasha and her husband were second on the list for adoption, so they removed themselves from the list to make room for someone else. Then, at 12 weeks, she started to bleed profusely. She was hysterical. Fortunately, it was a common (but frightening) condition called a subchorionic hematoma that usually resolves itself. Blood had pooled between the chorion, a membrane surrounding the embryo, and the uterine wall, and her uterus was expelling it. Thankfully, it successfully resolved, but it was terrifying. No more heavy lifting for Natasha!

She carried to term and delivered a huge healthy baby boy with white-blond hair and bright blue eyes, whom she named Henry. Her husband jokingly wondered where such a blond baby came from because they were both brunettes. Henry was a perfect and happy baby. Natasha's dream had materialized, and her family was complete. After delivery, she had an IUD put in.

She sold all their baby stuff, and she and Anthony embraced the contentment of a family of four. When Henry was 15 months old, she had her IUD removed because it kept slipping and was uncomfortable. She didn't give it another thought.

A few weeks later, she was listening to a Martina McBride Christmas song on the radio, and she burst into tears. Natasha wasn't a crier, so she wondered what was wrong. Was she stressed out and hadn't realized it? Was something else bothering her? Then it dawned on her that it had been six weeks since her last period, and she could've mistaken pregnancy symptoms for what she thought was a mild flu. It had never occurred to her that she might be pregnant again. On Christmas Eve, as they were preparing for the next morning, she took five pregnancy tests, because she could not believe that she was pregnant. All were immediately positive. Each time she stared at the test results in disbelief.

Natasha was nervous about breaking the news to Anthony. He had been sitting by the Christmas tree sipping a seasonal ale, marveling that they would soon be getting their lives back. They could now go camping and rock climbing again, since their kids were four-and-a-half years and fifteen-months old. Natasha decided to let him enjoy the feeling of freedom from babyhood a little bit longer.

The next day, Natasha told Anthony she had some big news.

"Please tell me you're pregnant, because last night I dreamed we had three kids," he said.

"You're kidding me?" She showed him the tests, and they went to their midwife immediately. She was already 12 weeks pregnant! She had apparently been between six and eight weeks pregnant during the IUD removal. Thankfully, her baby was unharmed. The pregnancy and delivery went smoothly, and baby Keegan was born healthy.

Natasha was confused about her dream. Anthony had dreamt about three kids, but she had only seen two. After trying to recreate the old dream in her mind, she decided that she must have been pregnant with Keegan in the dream while Charlotte was in her lap, obscuring the pregnancy.

Reflecting on her fertility journey, having experienced everything from a planned adoption to an unplanned pregnancy,

Natasha concluded that everything happens for a reason. She advises friends to have faith—everything that is supposed to happen is going to happen. She's an enthusiastic advocate for adoption and feels it's a wonderful gift for all involved.

When Natasha was pregnant with Henry, some people would say in front of her young daughter, "You'll love the biological baby more than the adopted one."

"I don't see how that's possible," Natasha replied.

She feels that, despite Charlotte's Korean heritage, she fits in perfectly and actually looks the most like them, because their boys are so fair-haired. Charlotte isn't her second choice or her second-best child. She is her firstborn child and one of the three loves of her life. Where other people see race, all she sees is the face of the child she loves.

She tells Charlotte, "Most babies come from their mommy's tummy, but you came from my heart."

Natasha feels there is a child for all of us. No matter how bleak it may seem at times, life has a way of working out if we just let it happen. It may not look the way we expect, but it will be more beautiful than we could have imagined.

SURROGACY: WOMB FOR RENT

Giving up one's body for nine months to help another woman achieve her dream of motherhood is another one of the most selfless things a woman can do. Surrogates, while compensated for their service, give the gift of their bodies for nine months to gestate and deliver someone else's baby. Most surrogates earn around $25,000 base pay, plus all medical and legal expenses, prenatal vitamins, maternity clothes, childcare, meals, and other pregnancy-related expenses, even acupuncture if needed. Some women opt for altruistic surrogacy, meaning they don't get paid, except for expenses. This is usually to help a friend or family member who can't carry her own child.

Sometimes, women become surrogates for strangers because they understand the pain and heartache of infertility. One surrogate learned how her own parents endured infertility nightmares to have her and her brother, and that drove her to offer her womb for rent. She carried twins for a couple and said that for her surrogacy felt like "carrying someone else's dreams."[5]

---

5. Carrying 'Dreams': Why Women Become Surrogates, All Things Considered, April 17, 2012, Marisa Penaloza.

A BEAUTIFUL ARRANGEMENT

Dahlia came in for treatment in April of 2016, after trying to conceive for two long years. Battle-weary and discouraged, she shared that she had suffered three miscarriages, each happening somewhere between six and eight weeks. After her third miscarriage, she figured it was time to see a fertility doctor. She was hopeful when he explained she had a uterine septum, a common cause of miscarriage. He surgically removed the septum, and Dahlia thought, Maybe this time my pregnancy will take.

Dahlia and her husband, Forrest, tried a few more times, and three times, her fertilized eggs stopped short of becoming babies. Their hearts broke with each attempt. They concluded the uterine septum wasn't the problem. But what was? Dahlia wasn't ready to give up. Not yet.

The reproductive endocrinologist ran blood tests, checking genetics and clotting factors. All of Dahlia's tests came back normal. The doctor was at a loss: "Sorry. I wish I could be more helpful."

"I've been thinking about trying acupuncture," Dahlia said.

"Sure. Why not? What do you have to lose?"

Dahlia jumped up on the treatment table and reclined. I took her hand in mine, felt her pulses, then walked around the table, and took the other. When I asked, she complained of lower back pain, night sweats, excessive warmth during the day, trouble staying asleep, and having to get up to pee many times during the night.

The quality of her Chinese Kidney pulses paired with her symptoms above indicated Yin deficiency with internal heat. She had virtually every symptom of Yin deficiency. When I asked to see her tongue, she produced a peeled, geographic tongue, with patches of tongue coating missing. Western medicine views this as normal, but Chinese medicine sees this as an indication of Yin deficiency.

To tonify her Yin and remedy the situation, I started Dahlia on herbs to cool her body. This helped her sleep and eventually cooled her down, though it took time. Her periods became lighter with fewer clots and minor cramps.

After four months of acupuncture and herbs, Dahlia became pregnant! She didn't have many symptoms, but this is typical of some pregnancies. At seven weeks, she had brown clotting, which alarmed her, but on the ultrasound, the baby's heartbeat was normal, as was the size of the fetus. Did Dahlia dare to hope? Dare to dream?

I put her on Chinese herbs designed to stop bleeding during pregnancy, which worked. But she still felt overheated and was hot to the touch. Was there some sort of autoimmune issue causing her internal heat, a sign of inflammation?

Once again, around eight weeks, Dahlia lost her baby. She was deeply disheartened and decided to shift her focus away from trying to conceive.

When Dahlia returned to treatment six months later, she complained of aches and pains. "Not only am I training for a half-marathon; I was also in an accident with a bus."

"Oh, geez! Are you okay?"

"Yes, just minor whiplash and back strain."

"It's never a dull moment with you."

She laughed. "I know. I thought taking a break from the baby train would give me some much-needed R&R."

I laughed. "I love running, but training for a half-marathon doesn't sound like relaxing to me!"

"No kidding!" Dahlia said.

"Speaking of the baby train, are you hopping back on?" I asked.

She shook her head. "Thinking about it now, maybe not. It might be time to consider a whole different tack."

"Oh? What's that?" I asked.

"It makes me sad to give up, but I don't know how much more I can handle. After seven miscarriages with no explanation, it might be time for a surrogate."

"In my mind, that's not giving up at all."

She came in once every three to six months for neck and shoulder pain, but never again for fertility.

Dahlia and her husband chose traditional surrogacy, where the carrier is also the egg donor. This more old-fashioned approach doesn't involve IVF but is instead done through intra-uterine insemination (IUI). Traditional surrogacy is not used that much anymore, as the surrogate can understandably become attached to her genetic child. May, their surrogate, wasn't interested in having another child of her own and really wanted to help them. Dahlia and May formed a deep friendship, even though they lived in different states.

I was curious about their friendship, so I asked, "What's it like to have a surrogate in your life?"

Dahlia said, "Thanks to my support group and therapist, I was genuinely fine with someone else carrying my baby. What I really wanted was to be a mom, and I certainly tried very hard to do it myself, but it wasn't in the cards. I'm so grateful that May was willing to give us such a generous gift so that Forrest and I could be parents."

They found an OB/GYN who was willing to perform the IUI. Forrest made his donation when the surrogate was ovulating, and the doctor performed the insemination. It didn't work the first time but did on the second try!

People today are much more likely to choose gestational surrogacy, where the surrogate is just the carrier and not genetically related to the baby. It's legally much safer for the intended parents. But after all Dahlia had gone through, she was not interested in going through a medication-intensive egg retrieval. This meant the child wouldn't be genetically related to her, but she was okay with it. She didn't want to subject her body to more fertility drugs or surgeries. May also preferred traditional surrogacy because it meant fewer drugs for her.

Traditional surrogacy is legally complicated, so it's a risky path and not allowed in some states. Fortunately, May lived in a surrogacy-friendly state. In many states, the baby must first be put up for adoption and the intended parents then adopt it. This state allowed them to have a pre-birth order that declared the baby legally theirs even before she was born. Dahlia and Forrest signed the pre-birth order the day before their baby shower, which was a lovely omen. According to the couple's attorney, this process was fortunate and quite unusual. Had they done the surrogacy in Colorado, they would have had to adopt the baby, complete a home study, and endure all the rigamarole of formal adoption.

I loved treating Dahlia and following the progress of her daughter's growth inside the surrogate. I continued to treat Dahlia for anxiety and neck and shoulder pain up until her daughter was born. The surrogate gave birth to Azalea, a healthy, happy little girl, and her parents couldn't be happier.

During our final session, Dahlia shared more details about her relationship with her surrogate.

"May and I have a good relationship. We consider her family part of ours! After she gave birth to Azalea, we had a lovely heart-to-heart about what we had been through—the many conversations with lawyers and social workers, the contract, two rounds of IUI, the pregnancy, the pre-birth order, and the C-section. If you go through so much with someone, you're definitely bonded forever."

PREGNANCY AND INFANT LOSS: WHEN THINGS GO WRONG

The stories in this section come with a trigger warning. They are not all happy, nor are they all hopeful. Sometimes fertility journeys take twists and turns into the darkest places imaginable.

Infant and child loss is one of the most painful things a woman can ever experience. Children are not supposed to die before their parents, but tragically, it happens. Sometimes babies are snatched up by the hand of fate just days after making their grand entrance into the world. Sometimes they don't even make it into the world at all.

The women featured in these stories are incredibly courageous; they persevered after the worst thing imaginable happened. Not only that, but they are also brave enough to share their stories.

EVERY PART OF MY SOUL

The first time Michelle came to my office, she was 36½ weeks pregnant with her second child, Leigh. She had no problem getting pregnant with either of her children, the older of which was a three-year-old son named Jenson.

Because of her "advanced maternal age" (she was almost 41 years old), the OB/GYN wanted to induce her at 39 weeks. According to studies, the risk of stillbirth after 40 doubles from one in 1,000 to two in 1,000 between 39 and 40 weeks of pregnancy. These are low odds, but if it happens to you, the odds are 100 percent. Nobody wants to live through that.

Michelle wanted to get the ball rolling naturally, so she came in for pre-birth acupuncture, which has been shown to decrease the amount of time in labor. It relaxes the pelvic floor and cervix, as well as the mom-to-be.

At 36½ weeks, Michelle was already 2.3 cm dilated. Michelle came in twice, and about 36 hours after her second treatment, Leigh was born healthy at 38 weeks. I never expected to see Michelle or her interesting back tattoos again.

Michelle came to see me again just over a year later. I ushered her into my office and said, "How's little Leigh?"

When she tearfully glanced toward the window, a knot seized my gut. I hoped I was reading too much into her body language.

"Well, that's just it." She couldn't meet my gaze. "She didn't make it."

"What?" I couldn't stop my tears, but I throttled the sob wedged in my throat. "Michelle, I…"

"You don't have to say anything to comfort me. I know it's so hard to talk about. I mean, it's one of the most unthinkable things any parent can experience."

I was amazed by her strength and resolve. She was holding it together so much better than I. "What happened?" When the words came tumbling out of my mouth, I wished I could retrieve them. "If you'd rather not talk about it, I understand."

"I don't mind. My baby girl died of Sudden Infant Death Syndrome at just over three months old. One morning when I went to her crib to feed and change her, she wasn't breathing. I stared at her and willed her to breathe. I was afraid to touch her because I knew if she were cold, I'd have lost her. I let out a wail that could have been heard all over town. Every part of my soul was shattered."

I could only imagine how much courage Michelle had mustered to return to my office. The last time she'd been in, she was excited about delivering Leigh. I'd heard people say, "If I lost a child, I don't think I could ever try again." Admittedly, I was probably one of those people. But to my surprise, I had seen more than one patient try to get pregnant right after losing a child.

Michelle had been working with a fertility clinic and had already gone through one round of IVF at the end of October. It had produced only two embryos, both of which were chromosomally abnormal. The clinic suggested she take supplements for egg health as well as try acupuncture. That's when she summoned up the courage to return.

Michelle came in twice a week for five months before her retrieval. Each treatment was emotionally fraught for Michelle. So many questions tortured her. *What if it worked? Would she be trying to replace Leigh? How could she ever replace her?* But the worst question of all was *What if it didn't work?*

This time the clinic retrieved ten eggs, which produced only one embryo. It was sent off for pre-implantation genetic testing. One very good grade AA embryo came back. While it was an amazing feat that at 43, Michelle had produced one perfect embryo, it was also intensely stressful; all her eggs were literally in one basket.

The old questions arose. *What if it worked? What if it didn't work?* She made peace with the questions, reminding herself that her body and uterus knew very well how to be and stay pregnant. Six months after restarting acupuncture, the clinic transferred the embryo into her uterus.

During her six months of acupuncture, Michelle also began seeing my husband, Scott, for energy work. He has been an acupuncturist for as long as I have, and we practice together. But he has progressed over time into an energy healer after taking two years of coursework in advanced energy healing. Three months into acupuncture treatment, Michelle saw him weekly to clear any energetic blockages that may have remained after losing Leigh. Scott saw the energetic remains of Leigh's umbilical cord in Michelle's uterus, as well as scar tissue around her heart. He cleared these up energetically over the course of many treatments. By the end of his treatments, he saw that her uterus was healed up, though the scar tissue around her heart remained. She loved the energy work and felt it helped immensely.

Seven months after restarting acupuncture and two weeks after the embryo transfer, Michelle was pregnant again! She was thrilled but also very emotional. It still didn't feel real, and anxiety prevailed, as so much was out of her control. When the unthinkable happens, you know anything is possible. Your innocence is lost. But Michelle tried not to dwell there and instead focused on a positive outcome.

At seven and a half weeks, she began bleeding and even passed some tissue. She called me to say that the baby looked good on the ultrasound but there was a large subchorionic hematoma at the base of her uterus. According to her doctor, this was not uncommon in women who have had IVF, specifically a frozen embryo transfer, who were of advanced maternal age, and who had had more than one baby. So, basically, just like Michelle. Fortunately, the baby had implanted high in her uterus, in the best possible place, away from the hematoma.

The RE took her off the baby aspirin she was taking to prevent the hematoma from worsening. The spotting slowed down and became old blood. She was put on bed rest, as the RE was concerned about the size of the hematoma. Michelle continued to see me for acupuncture, shuffling carefully into the office in her pajamas and slippers so as not to disturb the precious cargo in her uterus. I saw her until she reached 13 weeks.

I texted Michelle when she was seven months pregnant to see how she was doing.

She texted: *Baby is fine! It was a hard three months from October to December, since that's when Leigh was alive. I chose to really focus my thoughts on her for that period. I felt she deserved my attention. I'm getting a doula so she can help me navigate sadness and joy before and after birth. I'm trying to be joyful every day—it can be hard sometimes. I'm really looking forward to starting treatments with you again soon! It feels very close actually, only two months, and then we're really ready for baby to be here with us. I feel movement every day, getting stronger and more consistent. We're at the doc's every 2 weeks, which makes me feel better to hear the baby's heartbeat. Feeling a little better each day!"*

The next time I heard from Michelle was after her baby girl, Claire had been born. At 33 weeks, Michelle was at work and began experiencing contractions. She didn't think it could really be time, as it was still too early in the pregnancy. However, in the middle of the night, it was intense enough to keep her awake, and the contractions were closer together. At the hospital, the OB saw that Michelle was already dilated to 9cm, so they got her ready for delivery. The epidural didn't work (!), so she was put completely under anesthesia and prepared for a C-section. This turned out to be fortunate, as Claire was breech, or butt down, and her umbilical cord was wrapped around her neck. While Michelle was in recovery, her husband was able to be with the baby in the NICU.

As of the writing of this story, baby Claire is in the NICU, off supplemental oxygen and exceeding expectations. She looks just like her big sister, Leigh, with the same eyes, same nose, and same yawn. Michelle wrote, "It's hard to be back in a medically fragile space again. My trauma response says it will look the same as it did for Leigh, even though everyone tells me she's doing so well. I would have felt cheated, I think, if she were a boy or somehow didn't look like her. It makes me feel like Leigh is connected to us through her. I'm grateful to see her again in a new body."

UNBROKEN COURAGE

Alicia, a 28-year-old teacher, sat down, clasped her hands, and said, "Are you ready for some drama?"

I had seen so much over my years as an acupuncturist; I figured I would be nonplussed no matter what she shared with me. "Sure," I said.

"It's super creepy."

"Try me."

"So, when I was fourteen, I had intense pain in my lower abdomen—so intense it made me vomit. Then one day, I passed out. My mom took me to the ER, and they discovered I had a nine-pound dermoid cyst on my right ovary. Nine pounds. Can you imagine?"

I shook my head. *That's the weight of a baby.*

"It had split open, and I was bleeding internally. Fortunately, they were able to save the ovary and fallopian tube, and oh—my life. I might have been a goner."

A dermoid cyst is a growth that develops when skin becomes trapped during fetal development. This kind of cyst can exist in the sinuses, brain, spinal cord, and on the ovaries. When the cyst is on an ovary and develops during a young woman's reproductive years, it can grow skin, teeth, and hair.

When Alicia came to see me, she and her husband had been trying to conceive for three years. She had PCOS, and her husband had low sperm motility. Also, she had scar tissue on her right fallopian tube from her cyst surgery, which prevented the egg from going down the tube on the right side. The cards were stacked against them. They had tried two IUIs, but every time she grew multiple cysts with Clomid, so they had to stop trying this method. They moved on to IVF.

IVF is expensive, and since both of them are teachers, Alicia and her husband weren't rolling in cash. To save money, she and her husband took part in a study in which retrieved eggs were matured in a dish instead of inside the body, as in a typical IVF cycle. With their fertility doctor's help, they had retrieved 14 eggs two months earlier and matured them in a dish. Using this method, only four eggs matured, and just one fertilized. Alicia came to see me to prepare for her frozen embryo transfer.

She had elevated Doppler readings in one of her uterine arteries, indicating that blood flow to the uterus on that side was restricted, so her fertility doctor sent her in for electroacupuncture prior to transfer. The uterine arteries feed the uterus and ovaries, and if the flow of blood in them is impeded, or restricted, fertility and IVF outcomes aren't as good. Studies show electroacupuncture is effective in improving the blood flow, so many fertility doctors send patients to acupuncturists for this procedure. Studies also show that two treatments per week for the four weeks leading up to embryo transfer is most effective.

Alicia came in for the prescribed eight treatments, and she got pregnant! Remember in the movie, *Finding Nemo* when all the fertilized fish eggs were eaten by a barracuda except for the one that became Nemo? They named their embryo "Nemo," since it was the only one to survive the IVF. However, even after hearing Nemo's heartbeat during ultrasounds at six and eight weeks, she miscarried between nine and ten weeks. Alicia and her husband were devastated. They took a break for several months to heal emotionally and physically, got healthy, and returned for more acupuncture.

Alicia had changed fertility doctors, and she and her husband decided to try another IUI cycle with Letrozole and Menopur instead of Clomid. This time, there were no cysts, and she had two big eggs. Her husband's sperm count was within normal limits for an IUI. Everything looked great! But again, it didn't work. A few months later, she came back to prepare for another IVF, this time a fresh cycle with a new clinic. She chose to do ten acupuncture treatments before her transfer. This was useful for Alicia because she experienced many side effects from the drugs, including hot flashes, bloating, and weepiness, which acupuncture helped ameliorate. She was understandably nervous, as she had had such a rough road trying to conceive, and the acupuncture helped her to feel calm.

This cycle, she responded very well, and they retrieved 30 eggs! Fourteen fertilized and seven embryos made it to day four. They transferred two, and Alicia became pregnant with twins! She and her husband were over the moon.

Alicia needed an emergency cerclage at 20 weeks, as her cervix was becoming too short to hold the twins inside. In a cerclage, a cervix is sewed closed to keep the babies in. In an unbelievably tragic turn of events unrelated to the cerclage, her daughter Cora died in her womb at 22 weeks. She was devastated. Adding insult to injury, Alicia was diagnosed with pre-eclampsia at 28 weeks. Her doctor ordered bed rest until 37 weeks. She also had severe gestational diabetes that she controlled with diet and medicine.

Alicia called me a week after her delivery. "My delivery was the most surreal day of my life. Can you imagine experiencing heaven and hell at the same time?" she said.

"No; no, I can't."

"I mean, I welcomed into the world my little Idan—pink, wiggly, crying up a storm, and of course the cutest little bundle of love. And then…his sister, Cora. The sister he would never know."

She abruptly stopped talking, and I only heard heaving breath and sniffles. "Sorry, I don't mean to… Cora wasn't given a chance. My sister and husband saw her bundled in a pink blanket and we had photos taken. She had brown wisps of hair. They also had close-up shots of her hands and feet. I couldn't bring myself to hold her, and I regret that so much." Her sniffles gave way to sobbing.

"It's okay. It's heartbreaking—nothing any parent should ever go through."

After delivery, the medical team determined that Cora had had an "umbilical cord accident" shutting off oxygen to her little body. They determined it was due to insufficient Wharton's jelly in her cord. Wharton's jelly lubricates the inside of the cord to keep it from kinking and causing cord accidents.

When Idan was 14 months old, Alicia experienced sharp pelvic pain that doubled her over, so she had an ultrasound. They found three cysts on her left ovary and told her that she had ovulated. Two weeks later, Alicia and her husband found out they were pregnant naturally! She had low progesterone and went on progesterone supplements to support the pregnancy. She was also extremely nauseous and had to take Zofran to control it.

At the ten-week ultrasound, her doctor said her baby looked "a little different" but was measuring on track. At the 13-week appointment to recheck the baby, they found that the baby boy was missing an arm, had a large nuchal fold (a sign of chromosomal abnormalities), underdeveloped legs, was missing a femur, and his pelvis was backward. The doctor told them that if they continued with the pregnancy, it would be dangerous for Alicia, the boy would need to have his legs amputated, and if he survived, he would be wheelchair-bound.

Considering the trauma she already had been through, this was beyond awful. Alicia and her husband made the near-impossible decision to have a dilation and evacuation (D&E) at 18 weeks; this was not a decision they took lightly. She named her son "Tyr" after the Norse god who sacrificed his right hand to save the world.

One week after the procedure, she was bleeding heavily, and the doctor determined that she had excessive scar tissue, causing issues. Without anesthesia or a numbing agent, the clinic performed a D&C (dilation and curettage). She wished she had stopped them because the pain was off the charts! She later found out that the D&C created more damage. Alicia spent the summer in extreme pain, trying to determine the source. She went to two doctors and the emergency room, and they all thought it was "in her head" because the ultrasounds didn't show anything.

She went back to her fertility doctor, a pelvic pain specialist, who did an HSG, a procedure where dye is pushed through the fallopian tubes to check for patency and determined there was a blockage in one of them. To investigate further, he performed a laparoscopy and found that her ovary was twisted, a "chocolate" cyst (an ovarian cyst filled with blood) had grown on it, and another cyst had ruptured. All were embedded in scar tissue attached to her uterus. He then did a more serious surgery, removing her ovary and fallopian tube on that side, and a section of her upper uterus. Her doctor advised to wait at least six to nine months to heal before trying for another child.

Alicia summoned immense courage and came back to see me a year later at age 33 to prepare for another embryo transfer. Understandably, she was nervous about it. She was unable to continue that IVF cycle because she had ovulated, even while on ovulation-suppressing drugs. The next month she came back, and we did electroacupuncture again. This time ovulation was successfully suppressed, and the doctor transferred one embryo. The pregnancy ended in a chemical pregnancy, one in which a positive pregnancy test just as quickly turns negative before 5 weeks gestation.

Alicia and her husband do not give up easily, so they did one more frozen embryo transfer, and she became pregnant with her son, Cohen. The doctors put in a preventative cerclage which held through the whole pregnancy. She had a partial placental abruption at 24 weeks when she unexpectedly had to break up a fight at school. The baby was unharmed, but she was put on bed rest. The pre-eclampsia she experienced in her twin pregnancy returned at

24 weeks, and again she suffered from severe gestational diabetes. She was on total bed rest until 37 weeks.

Cohen's birth was scheduled, but Alicia was in the hospital the week leading up to the C-section because of her diabetes and high blood pressure. Even though Cohen's umbilical cord was wrapped around his neck twice, the delivery was so much easier than the twins'. The recovery was okay, but the whole family got the stomach flu three days later. Alicia also endured a bout of postpartum anxiety and started therapy. She is still on anti-anxiety meds after being diagnosed with PTSD, OCD, and anxiety. Thankfully, it is managed and today Alicia is feeling good.

Alicia has two healthy, happy boys and says it was worth every single second. From start to finish, Alicia and her husband spent eight years to have two living children.

She loves every one of her five children—Nemo, twins Cora and Idan, Tyr, Jude, and Cohen. The family created a remembrance garden in their backyard. Cora has a tree, Tyr has a birdhouse, a rose bush and an angel statue, and Nemo has a little gold star. For Christmas every year, they get Tyr and Cora small ornaments.

Alicia told me the story of Cora's tree. "The year after Cora passed, we went to a nursery to find her tree. As I walked around, I became increasingly sad. Then there it was—a beautiful fire maple. I sat under the tree and sobbed. The poor workers were so confused. We brought the lovely red tree home and planted it and later placed a beautiful plaque underneath.

"In 2017, we decided to move. The only thing that stopped me was Cora's tree. I prayed she would give us permission to go.

"A month before we left, my husband found three saplings under her tree. We put the saplings into three little pots. One survived and we kept it in our kitchen window for over a year. Amazingly, the tree survived! When we planted it the summer of 2018, it was only a two-inch sapling and boy, did it take off! I believe Cora communicated that it was okay to move, and she came with us.

"My husband made a little shelter to protect Cora's tree. It was so tiny at first, and we were afraid summer storms with hard-driving hail might kill it, but it grew a foot last summer. I believe it is Cora still with us."

OVARIAN REBELLION

Annie first came to see me in 2012 when she was just 26 years old. Annie was a true Western gal with long auburn curls, dressed in Cruel Girl jeans and Ariat cowboy boots. Lovely and thoughtful, if I asked her a question, she always asked about me in return. Even though she was the focus in the treatment room, it's always lovely to spend time with someone who wants to know how you are doing.

Eager to be a mother, she and her husband, Caleb, had been trying to conceive for over two years. Annie had been going to a local fertility doctor for a year, and was diagnosed with anovulation, the failure to ovulate regularly. The go-to treatment for this is Clomid, an oral medication used to treat female infertility. After three months of Clomid, Annie still didn't ovulate, which was very unusual. She was dealing with some stubborn ovaries!

Annie learned that she had celiac disease, an inability to tolerate gluten, so she eliminated all the comfort food—pasta, pizza, and bread—from her diet. She quickly lost 13 pounds and got her period. This confirmed something Chinese medicine has known for centuries—that for many women, diet has a profound effect on fertility and menstrual cycles. Progress at last!

I treated Annie by supporting her digestion and attempting to promote ovulation naturally. Although she was healthy with a normal BMI, she had been diagnosed with PCOS. I treated her with electroacupuncture over her ovaries. This is a form of acupuncture where a small electric current is gently passed between pairs of needles. It may sound painful, but it is, in fact, very relaxing. The added stimulation over the ovarian points helps promote ovulation.

Because Annie lived three hours away in Wyoming, she only came in for treatment every two weeks. We both looked forward to her treatments so we could catch up on each other's lives. In her eternally positive and cheerful way, she described how she was fixing up her house and she planned to talk her husband into a farm that had at least one miniature animal of each kind—a donkey, a horse, and a pig. She already had a miniature Australian shepherd, so she was on her way.

After seven months, the biweekly acupuncture and powerful herbs didn't help her ovulate. So, Annie went back to the fertility doctor. She had a couple of menstrual cycles, which was an improvement, but her end goal wasn't a period. It was a baby!

The fertility doctor found that Annie had plenty of follicles, but they were not interested in ovulating. They were staging an ovarian rebellion. Acupuncture and herbs improve egg health and balance out the hypothalamic-pituitary-ovarian (HPO) axis to regulate menstrual cycles as evidenced by the fact that Annie had a couple of periods in the seven months we worked together. However, sometimes acupuncture and herbs are not enough, and Western medicine is the push needed to make ovulation happen. The fertility doctor put her on Letrozole, an ovulation-stimulating drug, to trigger ovulation, and it worked right away.

At long last, Annie was pregnant!

Her pregnancy progressed nicely, even though she discovered she had placenta previa—a condition in which the placenta sits on top of the cervix. This can be dangerous to the child and the mother. When the cervix opens in labor, it can cause the placenta to tear away from the uterine wall, triggering bleeding. If a woman starts bleeding uncontrollably, an emergency C-section must be performed to save the baby's and mother's lives.

When Annie was 31 weeks pregnant with her son, her placenta spontaneously ruptured, which allowed infection to permeate her uterine lining, not to mention profuse bleeding. Annie was life-flighted from the hospital in Wyoming to one in Denver with a high-level NICU. Trigg James was born by emergency C-section on November 1, 2013, at just 31 weeks gestation. He was 18.5 inches long and weighed 3 lbs. 13 oz. He fought hard to survive, and the doctors worked mightily to save him, but he died due to major organ failure and a massive pulmonary embolism on November 3. Annie and her husband were devastated. They leaned into their faith and grieved for their son.

When the couple came in for Annie's first treatment after Trigg died, we sat together.

"He was perfect, but we must accept that God had a different plan," Caleb said.

Annie pulled out her phone and showed me photos. "Look at him. Isn't he beautiful?"

He wore a knitted yellow hat and was wired up in the NICU. "He's so precious."

"Our son only graced the planet for forty-eight hours before rejoining God," Annie said and could not hold back the tears. Caleb held her and cried with her.

I am a reluctant crier, but tears flowed down my cheeks as I felt the weight of their profound loss and witnessed their raw grief.

Incredibly brave, after a year and a half, Annie moved forward with more Letrozole and other fertility drugs to assist in getting pregnant. The fertility doctors performed between nine and eleven medicated IUIs over two years. Generally, fertility doctors stop performing IUIs after three to five tries. However, since Annie's body was so resistant to ovulating, and since it had worked in the past, they kept trying.

During an appointment in October, Annie told me that she and Caleb were traveling to San Diego to honor Trigg's second birthday with a balloon release over the Pacific Ocean. I felt her pulse and suspected that she was pregnant. I shared my hunch with her. She was thrilled and couldn't wait to get home to take a pregnancy test. Her pulses hadn't lied, and indeed, she was! However, in another unfair blow, that pregnancy was short-lived. Life was once again unkind to this lovely couple.

After taking some much-needed time to recover, Annie and Caleb decided to move forward with IVF in January of 2016. A little over two years after Trigg's birthday, they began. Young and healthy and typical of women with PCOS, Annie produced many follicles. In one of the most impressive cases I'd seen, Annie produced 50 eggs! Thirty of those fertilized, and 22 embryos were very good. The final embryo count: 13 of the highest quality. Amazingly, Annie did not suffer from ovarian hyperstimulation syndrome

(OHSS). She had the bloating, distended belly, and ovarian pain characteristic of OHSS, but she did not retain fluid or have any blood clots or problems breathing, thank goodness. She had been through enough!

Because of Annie's age and the high quality of her embryos, in addition to her past pregnancy history, she, her husband, and the doctor decided to transfer only one embryo. The risk of carrying twins was too high, and since her egg quality was so good, the chance of twins was also high. They wanted to maximize the safety of her next baby, and there can be prematurity and complications with twins.

Finally, at age 30, Annie was pregnant again! She suffered from nausea until the end of her first trimester. Gratefully, her placenta cooperated this time and was positioned away from her cervix. The baby measured perfectly, and her pregnancy went smoothly. Her second, darling son, Traegger, was born healthy on October 5.

Annie and Caleb had 12 excellent embryos remaining, so in March of 2018, they started the IVF process again. They transferred one embryo in April, but sadly, it didn't take, and she suffered a miscarriage at six weeks, five days before Mother's Day. They tried a third IVF in January of 2019 that also ended at six weeks, five days, on Annie's birthday. They transferred one more in October of 2020, which was unsuccessful, and then two in December of 2020. Those didn't make it, either.

Caleb and Annie aren't done building their family. After everything they've endured, Annie says it's agonizing when Traegger cries for a baby brother or sister. That hurts her the most. But she has come to realize that her fertility journey is more about being mentally ready—in the game and strong—than it is being physically ready.

Annie believes that God has a plan, and they just need to trust Him. They will try IVF again one day. When the time comes to try again, they will be ready. She has faith that their boy, Traegger, will one day have a baby brother or sister.

THE COURAGE TO TRY AGAIN

Elizabeth came for acupuncture treatment after having suffered two miscarriages, the first at thirteen weeks, the second closer to eight weeks. She was no stranger to loss; nevertheless, you can imagine her anxiety about getting pregnant again.

During her first visit, Elizabeth shared her story. She had already seen an RE and because blood clotting is a common cause of miscarriage, she was waiting for blood test results to reveal what kind of clotting issues she may have had. The RE was also checking to see if autoimmune issues could be at play.

Elizabeth was also diagnosed with PCOS—a hormonal imbalance that interferes with the growth and release of eggs from the ovaries. In short, if you don't ovulate, you can't get pregnant. The good news is that PCOS is treatable. Elizabeth also had terrible menstrual cramps, a lot of stress, and high anxiety. Again, all treatable with acupuncture.

The picture became even clearer to me when she shared her test results. The results showed that she had one copy of the gene for factor V Leiden (or factor "5" Leiden), a blood clotting disorder. Women who carry the factor V Leiden mutation have an increased tendency to develop blood clots during pregnancy or when taking estrogen. Since Elizabeth had only one copy of the gene, it wasn't too severe, but she needed to take baby aspirin daily to thin her blood to improve her chances of implantation. If she became pregnant, she would need to inject a blood thinner called Lovenox from the time of the first pregnancy test to just before delivery. The blood thinner would reduce the chance of miscarriage due to blood clotting, as long as the embryo was genetically normal.

Along with acupuncture to boost egg health and help with anxiety, Elizabeth took Letrozole to encourage an egg to develop. Now here's the good news: three months after starting acupuncture and using Letrozole, she became pregnant, and her HCG (pregnancy hormone) was doubling normally every 48 hours to 90, 190, and 361 mIU/mL, respectively. She had all the signs and symptoms of pregnancy except for nausea, and at her six-week ultrasound, everything looked great. They saw a heartbeat, which calmed her anxiety a little.

With her history of miscarriages, Elizabeth was understandably very anxious she'd lose this baby, but by nine weeks, everything was going great. At ten weeks, bright red blood gushed out of her. The next day, it turned to old, brown blood and then gratefully, it stopped. The bleeding was caused by a subchorionic hematoma—blood pooled between the membrane surrounding the embryo and the uterine wall—that her uterus had eliminated in a natural but frightening manner. It was a terrifying experience, but, thankfully, her baby was fine. To deal with her intense anxiety, she saw me weekly, and every week, the "baby" pulse on her left wrist felt good and strong. Each wrist has three pulse positions on it that I feel for. The third position on the right side reveals the strength of Yang or progesterone. On the left side, the third position reveals the strength of the Yin, or what I call the "baby pulse."

At 12 weeks, she started vomiting from unknown causes and had an extra ultrasound to make sure everything was okay. The ultrasound showed a large blood clot on the baby's gestational sac. The RE instructed her to immediately stop the Lovenox injections and baby aspirin to prevent possible bleeding. The baby still looked great.

At 14 weeks, the blood clot was still there, but it was stable and possibly shrinking. She spotted dark brown blood. At 16 weeks, the baby measured perfectly on target. At long last, Elizabeth seemed to be out of the woods.

By 21 weeks of pregnancy, the clot had shrunk significantly, and her placenta wasn't affected by the clot. Blood clots on the placenta can be serious, causing miscarriage or stillbirth. I saw her at weeks 22, 25, 27, and 30. Elizabeth's pregnancy was going fine, though she was still anxious. At 30 weeks, her baby boy was big and healthy, and the clot on the gestational sac was nowhere to be seen.

At 35 weeks, she began to experience carpal tunnel symptoms in both wrists, a common symptom in late pregnancy, so I treated her for that. Acupuncture helps relieve the pain, but it unfortunately keeps coming back due to swelling from extra body fluid. The most effective solution for carpal tunnel in pregnancy is the delivery of the baby, but acupuncture does provide relief for several days. At 38 weeks, a year after starting treatment, she went in to deliver her son. Because he was in a transverse position, she had a C-section. But David was born healthy! Elizabeth had high blood pressure after delivery, so she was put on medicine to regulate it. To treat her persistent anxiety and pain in her arm, she came in for more acupuncture treatments.

Everything was going well for little David and his family. Days before he turned one, Elizabeth took David in for his one-year well-check appointment, part of which was a routine eye exam. The *InfantSEE®* program recommends all babies receive a baseline eye exam before they turn one. For years, Elizabeth had seen posters about it in her eye doctor's office, so it was on her radar, but many people have never heard of this recommendation or program.

During the exam, the doctor noticed something wasn't right but didn't know what it was. Elizabeth, her husband Dane, and David immediately were sent to a local pediatric ophthalmologist who confirmed something was wrong. That doctor referred them to a specialist in Denver at Children's Hospital. They had an in-office exam and—even without an eye exam which would have required sedation in a toddler—the specialist told them it was cancer: retinoblastoma. However, to be certain, and to learn more, David had his first exam under anesthesia days later at Children's Hospital.

With the cancer diagnosis confirmed, Elizabeth and Dane were devastated. This type of cancer develops rapidly from the immature cells of the retina, the light-detecting tissue of an eye. Almost half of children with retinoblastoma have a hereditary genetic defect associated with it. Most children lose their eye, but Elizabeth was determined to have David keep his.

To treat the tumor, she and her husband flew little David to a retinal cancer specialist in New York nine times in one year. The treatment included intra-arterial chemotherapy and laser.

Imagine taking a one-year-old on a plane back and forth to New York from Denver. Now imagine having to sedate him so he can be strapped to a table for chemotherapy and laser treatment in his affected eye. Nine times in one year!

Fortunately, after a year, David was completely cured and able to keep his eye. Through genetic testing, the family discovered that Elizabeth carries the RB1 microdeletion that caused David's retinoblastoma. There was a 50 percent chance that future children would inherit this same microdeletion. To avoid having to go through this trauma with another child, Elizabeth and her husband underwent IVF with preimplantation genetic diagnosis (PGD), so they could test the embryos and only use the ones free from the RB1 microdeletion. Retrieval and PGD constitute a very expensive and long process but knowing that she wouldn't have to go through the anxiety of possibly having another child with cancer was worth it. They ended up with nine chromosomally normal embryos.

Many months later, Elizabeth came to see me at 28 weeks pregnant with Alexander, a retinoblastoma-free baby boy. The first weeks of her pregnancy were good despite Elizabeth being cautious and nervous. Until roughly ten weeks, she felt a little more nauseous (no actual morning sickness) but didn't know if that was the pregnancy itself or the IVF hormones she was on. Overall, she mostly felt pure gratitude for being pregnant.

She had another subchorionic hematoma, like in her previous pregnancy, but fortunately, it never bled and resolved on its own.

This pregnancy had gone fairly well until her carpal tunnel symptoms flared up again. When she came to see me for symptom relief, I noticed her ankles were purple and swollen. The carpal tunnel symptoms barely went away with acupuncture this time, and she was miserable. I saw her at 31 weeks, 32 weeks, and the last time at 35 weeks of pregnancy.

A month later, I wrote her to check in with her. *Hi Elizabeth, I hope everything went well with your delivery. How are you doing?* A couple of hours later, I noticed her email in my inbox. I clicked on it, anxious to read Elizabeth's happy news. I hoped she included photos of her sweet baby boy.

Oh, Rachel, I have the worst news ever. On June 12th, I experienced a catastrophic uterine rupture and lost my baby. It's beyond devastating. I had a complete blood transfusion, was literally seconds from dying, and spent eight days in the hospital! My physical recovery will take longer than a regular C-section because of the trauma. I also have two DVTs (deep vein thrombosis) from the central line in my neck, massive swelling from all the fluids I received, etc.

Alexander was 7lbs, 10oz, 19.8 inches (a month early!) and totally perfect. I'm such a mess and so angry and heartbroken. Here are two pictures of my angel.

I stared at the screen, willing it to be different, willing Elizabeth's story to have a better outcome, willing life to be a little less brutal. Realizing I was holding my breath so I wouldn't feel the heartache, I reminded myself to breathe. As I did, tears cascaded down my cheeks. I was afraid to scroll down to see the photos, but I did out of respect for Elizabeth. Indeed, Alexander looked like a perfectly healthy baby, but with blue lips and fingernails. His beautiful face was perfectly formed, and his cheeks were chubby. *How was this fair? Why did she have to suffer so much to have a family?*

Elizabeth told me the story of the night Alexander was delivered.

"It all happened after tucking in David for bed. I felt a strange sharp pain and Alexander gave me a really hard kick. I dismissed the pains as contractions, given I was about 36 weeks along, but I progressively started feeling off. We called the clinic's after-hours nurse-line and were told, "It is probably dehydration, take some Tylenol and lie on your left side." I did as I was told, but things got worse because, every time I would sit up to hydrate, I blacked out. Each time I regained consciousness, I vomited. It happened several times and my husband later called the same after-hours line, told them what was happening, and they said I needed to go to the hospital right away. Because I could not physically sit up, we called 911. It was a strange mix of being lucid—aware of all the little details and sounds—and being so out of it. I recall quite a bit though, which is surprising given that I thought I was dying. Paramedics arrived, eventually strapped me to a board and whisked me off to the hospital. During the drive, they attempted at least ten locations all over my body to begin an IV but were unsuccessful because my blood pressure was too low. Little did we know that my entire abdomen was filled with blood. Dane woke up David (it was after midnight) and the two of them drove to the hospital."

A couple of months after recovering, Elizabeth came to see me for treatment of grief and residual pain from the DVTs in her arm and neck. I opened up grief points on her chest and arms with acupuncture so she could release more grief and sat with her as she cried. We talked about baby Alexander, about how alive he looked even though he was gone. We talked about how Elizabeth nearly died, and what that would have been like for her husband and son. She told me in tears that she was no longer allowed to bear children, as her uterus would surely rupture again. The doctors saved her uterus, but only for having periods—nothing else.

After some time had passed, a friend of Elizabeth's offered to carry her next baby as a surrogate. The legal documents were drawn up, and seven months after her catastrophic loss, one of Elizabeth and her husband's retinoblastoma-free embryos was transferred to her friend's uterus.

As grateful and hopeful as Elizabeth was, she had a tough time during the surrogate's pregnancy. She grieved for her lost baby Alexander. She grieved that she couldn't carry another child ever again. She struggled with excruciating PTSD from her previous experiences and with the fear of something bad happening during this pregnancy. Yet at the same time, she was so grateful for her amazing friend who was willing to donate her body for nine months to help Elizabeth build her family.

Elizabeth's third son, Grayson, was born in October of 2019. The pregnancy with Grayson was complication-free and his delivery went smoothly. Elizabeth said it was amazing being there and witnessing the entire thing—she thinks her friend is incredible. Although Elizabeth and her husband never saw Alexander with his eyes open, they can see Grayson's resemblance to Alexander, who lives on in his parents' hearts.

David adores his little brother, and the feeling is mutual! Elizabeth loves watching them interact and play. She is deeply grateful for her two healthy sons.

GLOSSARY

Western Medicine

AMH - Anti-Mullerian hormone (AMH) is a hormone secreted by cells in developing egg follicles. The level of AMH in a woman's blood is a good indicator of her ovarian reserve, or how many eggs are left. AMH does not change much during your cycle, so the blood sample can be taken at any time of the month. It is the most sensitive marker for ovarian reserve. AMH levels can vary depending on the lab used for testing, so it is best to use the same lab. Normal AMH levels are between 1 and 3 ng/mL. Lower than 1 indicates diminished ovarian reserve, while higher than 3 indicates polycystic ovaries (PCOS).

Antiphospholipid antibodies - Antiphospholipid antibodies (APA) are a group of immune proteins that the body produces against itself in an autoimmune response to phospholipids. APAs increase the risk of excessive blood clotting which can cause a developing embryo to miscarry. APAs can also contribute to pre-eclampsia. Treatment of APAs is with blood thinners once pregnant.

Balanced translocations - In a person with a balanced translocation, a piece of a chromosome is broken off and attached to another one in such a way that doesn't affect his or her development. However, when that person's cells divide to create an egg or sperm cells, they can end up with extra or missing genetic material, which can lead to miscarriage, depending on which chromosome and genes are affected.

Clomid - Clomid is an inexpensive method of ovulation induction. It is taken as a pill and it blocks estrogen receptors in the hypothalamus. The hypothalamus is then stimulated to release FSH and LH, since the hypothalamus senses that estrogen levels are low. This induces ovulation in a normal cycle. Clomid can cause decreased cervical mucus and a thin uterine lining. Clomid is also used by men who have a low sperm count and a low testosterone level. FSH increases sperm count, while LH increases testosterone.

D&C - Dilation and curettage (D&C), is a surgical procedure often performed after a first trimester miscarriage. In a D&C, dilation refers to opening the cervix, and curettage refers to removing the contents of the uterus. For some women, a D&C is a more physically comfortable way to pass the contents of a miscarriage.

Donor egg cycle - A donor egg cycle is an IVF cycle in which the eggs harvested are from another woman's ovaries. This is used when a woman wants to carry a pregnancy but cannot use her own eggs due to age-related fertility decline, genetic issues, or premature ovarian failure.

Donor sperm cycle - Donor sperm is used when the male partner has no sperm or a compromised semen analysis. It is also used when there is a genetic problem which could be inherited from the male. Single women and lesbian couples also may consider using donor sperm as a means to conceive.

Follistim - Follistim is the drug name for synthetic follicle-stimulating hormone (FSH). When injected, it helps a woman with healthy ovaries produce more eggs in a cycle. It can be used in IUI and IVF.

FSH - Follicle Stimulating Hormone (FSH) stimulates the growth and development of ovarian follicles. Your pituitary produces FSH until you ovulate. If you don't ovulate, your FSH levels will continue to rise. Your FSH level indicates how hard your body is working to ovulate. High levels are a sign of diminishing ovarian reserve (reduced egg numbers and lower egg quality). This hormone can vary greatly between cycles and can be misleading sometimes, since women with reduced ovarian reserve sometimes have a normal FSH level. It is not always useful in evaluating ovarian reserve and fertility potential.

HCG - Human chorionic gonadotropin (HCG) is a hormone secreted by the placenta during pregnancy which stimulates continued production of progesterone by the ovaries. HCG is also given as an injection to stimulate ovulation in controlled cycles.

HSG - Hysterosalpingogram (HSG) is a test that uses a dye and X-rays to confirm that the fallopian tubes are open, and that sperm can reach the egg.

Hysteroscopy - Hysteroscopy is the insertion of a scope into your uterus through the cervix to look for fibroids, scar tissue, a possible abnormal shape of the uterus, polyps, or any other issues that might be inside the uterus.

IUI - Intrauterine Insemination (IUI) is a procedure performed when semen that has been washed and concentrated is injected directly into the uterus. It is used for unexplained infertility, and in cases of poor sperm count or quality. It is also used when donor sperm is needed, a semen allergy exists, and when there are cervix/cervical mucus issues.

IVF - In Vitro Fertilization (IVF) is a procedure in which mature eggs are retrieved, then fertilized with sperm in a lab. In a fresh cycle, from the time of egg retrieval to embryo transfer into the uterus is 3-5 days. In a frozen cycle, the blastocysts are frozen for use at a later date, perhaps after genetic testing. There are many reasons one might utilize IVF, including unexplained infertility, missing or blocked fallopian tubes, sperm issues, advanced maternal age, and avoidance of genetic diseases.

Laparoscopy - Laparoscopy is the insertion of a laparoscope into the pelvic cavity through the abdominal wall to view the ovaries, fallopian tubes, and uterus for abnormalities. It is also used to check for and diagnose endometriosis. A laparoscopy is performed under general anesthetic and is a minimally invasive surgery.

Letrozole - Letrozole (aka Femara) is an estrogen-reducing anti-cancer drug used to induce ovulation. It decreases the total amount of estrogen in the body, causing the hypothalamus to release more FSH and LH, resulting in an ovulation. Letrozole doesn't thin the uterine lining or decrease cervical mucus.

LH - Luteinizing hormone (LH) in women is released by the anterior pituitary gland and it precedes ovulation. Ovulation predictor kits measure the release of LH, about 24-36 hours before ovulation. LH also stimulates the production of a corpus luteum to release progesterone. In men, LH stimulates production of testosterone.

Lovenox - Lovenox is an injectable blood-thinner used in pregnancy when women have blood-clotting issues that can cause miscarriage.

Menopur - Menopur is the drug name for follicle-stimulating hormone (FSH) plus luteinizing hormone (LH). It is natural in that it is collected from the urine of post-menopausal women, often nuns. It is injected to increase the number of follicles available for an IUI or IVF cycle.

NK (Natural Killer) cells - White blood cells that fight off viral-infected cells and tumors in the body. The research isn't clear at this time, but some researchers believe they are also involved in recurrent miscarriage.

Premature ovarian failure - Premature ovarian failure (POF) is the loss of normal function of ovaries before age 40. The ovaries don't produce normal amounts of estrogen or release eggs regularly, resulting in infertility.

Retrieval - Egg retrieval is when mature eggs are removed from the ovaries.

Septate Uterus - A deformity of the uterus which happens during fetal development. A membrane called the septum divides the uterus. This dividing septum is a fibrous band of tissue that doesn't supply the necessary nutrients to the developing embryo if the embryo implants onto the septum. Women with a septate uterus are at increased risk of miscarriage.

Subchorionic hematoma - The accumulation of blood within the folds of the chorion (the outer fetal membrane, next to the placenta) or between the uterus and the placenta itself. It can cause light to heavy spotting, but it may not. Most subchorionic bleeds resolve on their own and women go on to have healthy pregnancies.

Transfer - Embryo transfer is the last step in the IVF process when a fresh or frozen embryo is transferred via catheter to the mother's uterus.

Chinese Medicine

Blood stagnation - This is the number one cause of fertility issues that I see in my clinic. When blood stagnates, it can cause everything from painful cramps, to fibroids, to frequent miscarriages. Blood stagnation can cause tiny clots that cut off the blood supply to a developing embryo. Chinese herbs and other supplements thin the blood enough that blood stagnation can be addressed. Moving blood is tricky, as one could bleed too much, so *always* consult a trained herbalist before you take herbs, and *never* take them with blood-thinning medications. Do not prescribe these or other Chinese herbal formulas to yourself but consult a licensed acupuncturist instead.

Jiao - a section of the body according to Chinese medicine. The "lower Jiao" houses the reproductive organs and bladder. The "upper Jiao" houses the Heart and Lungs, while the "middle Jiao" houses the digestive organs.

Jing - Jing is the most important indicator of fertility. Jing is crucial for building teeth, bones, and eggs and sperm. Women and men with low reserves of Jing struggle with fertility issues because their eggs and sperm are poor quality. Jing is inherited from one's parents but is depleted with age, by drugs and from an unhealthy lifestyle. Jing deficiency can be turned around with months of herbs and acupuncture, but sometimes donor egg or sperm is needed.

Kidney Yin deficiency - A cause of low estrogen, Kidney Yin deficiency also manifests as a lack of cervical mucus. These women often are warm and sweaty at night, but not always. This takes time to reverse but responds nicely to fertility acupuncture and Chinese herbs.

Kidney Yang deficiency - Women who are cold in temperature, have low progesterone, and a low sex drive are low in Kidney Yang. This condition also responds nicely to fertility acupuncture and Chinese herbs and supplements.

Liver Qi stagnation - Liver Qi stagnation manifests as PMS and other hormonal imbalances. It responds beautifully to exercise, eliminating alcohol, and utilizing acupuncture and Chinese herbs. This is the easiest condition to treat because patients feel so much better after even a few minutes of receiving acupuncture.

Qi/Chi - Pronounced "Chee," Qi or Chi is the energy of the body. Each organ has its own type of Qi/Chi. Qi/Chi tends to get stuck or deficient, causing issues.

Spleen Qi deficiency - Women with this condition often bleed heavily during menstruation, sometimes extremely so. They can also suffer from fatigue, digestive issues, and miscarriages. I *always* treat the spleen, as it is the foundation for health in everyone. To treat your Spleen Qi (energy), step away from ice water, ice cream and large amounts of raw vegetables. Eat soups, roasted or steamed veggies, and drink warm beverages.

ACKNOWLEDGMENTS

In the two years that it took me to write these chapters, I had a lot of help. First, I want to thank my editor, Ann Tinkham, for improving these stories by suggesting and adding dialogue. Otherwise, they would have been very dry and not as easy to read. She has been my cheerleader throughout, and I am deeply grateful for her help. If you are reading this, go buy and read her books!

Thank you to everyone at Mark Graham Communications for agreeing this was a good idea for a book. Perhaps they say that to all potential clients, but I am grateful for their confidence and guidance.

Thank you to my friend and colleague, Maren Cahill, LAc, FABORM, for the support and cheerleading. I felt intimidated to publish this, worried that my super-intelligent colleagues might pass judgment on it, but her enthusiasm for this project helped me to proceed.

Thank you to my author friends, Corey Radman, Kelly Baugh, and Sarah Thompson, LAc, for advice and guidance and walks. I had no idea how much work went into writing a book. Go read their work, as well!

Thank you, Ellyn Dickmann, for reading the finished product from top to bottom when it was done and giving excellent advice. I really appreciate your generosity and constructive criticism.

Thank you, Jill Levine, for your cheerleading and friendship over the years. You really get what I do, and it's wonderful.

Thank you to my family for giving me space to write and hugs whenever I needed them. If I hadn't miscarried three times, I probably wouldn't have gone into fertility acupuncture, and Scott and I wouldn't have had these two awesome kids.

Most of all, thank you to my patients for agreeing to share their intimate, personal stories so that others might benefit from hearing them. You are reading their stories, but they lived through them.

ABOUT THE AUTHOR

Rachel Blunk, LAc, Fellow of the American Board of Oriental Reproductive Medicine (FABORM), is Northern Colorado's premier licensed and board-certified fertility acupuncturist. She is dedicated to helping women get pregnant and have a healthy pregnancy from start to finish.

A specialist in women's health and fertility acupuncture for over 20 years, she has helped hundreds of women get pregnant.

Having experienced her own struggle with fertility, Rachel provides the utmost in gentle and compassionate care. Patients feel listened to and understood, as well as confident in her techniques and in-depth knowledge of infertility treatments. Patients regain hope that conception is possible.

Rachel has attended the Integrative Fertility Symposium every year since its inception to learn the latest developments in fertility medicine. She also collaborates regularly with local Reproductive Endocrinologists, OB/GYNs and Nurse Midwives, helping women to get and stay pregnant.

Rachel is an avid outdoor enthusiast, business owner, wife, mother and now author. Join Rachel as she shares stories from two decades of caring for patients, helping them realize their dreams, meet their children, and change their lives in the most miraculous of ways.

You can follow her on Facebook at "Waiting on Pins and Needles." This book's website is www.WaitingOnPinsAndNeedles.com

RESOURCES

American Board of Oriental Reproductive Medicine (ABORM) www.ABORM.org

American Society for Reproductive Medicine (ASRM) www.ASRM.org

American Pregnancy Association www.AmericanPregnancy.org

American College of Obstetricians and Gynecologists (ACOG) www.ACOG.org

www.ingramcontent.com/pod-product-compliance
Lightning Source LLC
Chambersburg PA
CBHW052313220526
45472CB00001B/101